POWERSCULPT
FOR MEN

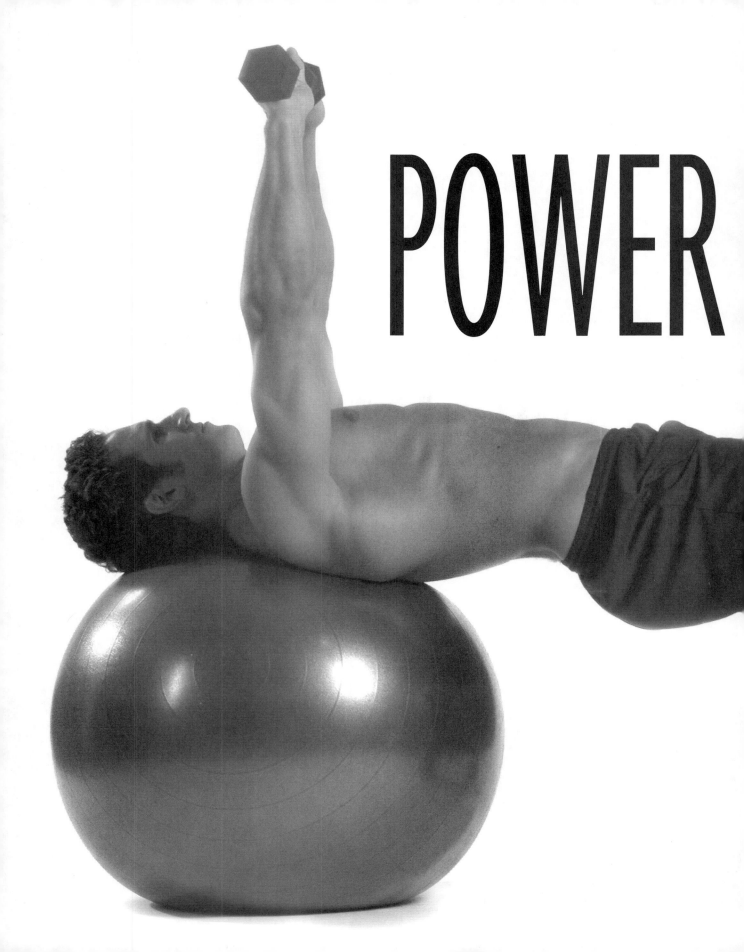

POWER

SCULPT FOR MEN

The Complete Body Sculpting & Weight Training Workout Using the Exercise Ball

By PAUL FREDIANI

PHOTOGRAPHS *by* PETER FIELD PECK

healthylivingbooks
NEW YORK · LONDON

A HEALTHY LIVING BOOK
Published by Hatherleigh Press
5-22 46th Avenue, Suite 200
Long Island City, NY 11101
Visit our Web site:
www.healthylivingbooks.com

Library of Congress Cataloging-in-Publication Data

Frediani, Paul, 1952-
PowerSculpt for men : the body sculpting & weight training workout using the exercise ball / by Paul Frediani ; photographs by Peter Field Peck.
     p. cm.
  Includes bibliographical references and index.
  ISBN 1-57826-181-3 (alk. paper)
  1. Exercise for men. 2. Weight training. 3. Swiss exercise balls. I. Title: Power sculpt. II. Title.
  GV482.5.F74 2004
  613.7'0449--dc22

                                        2004022263

Seek the advice of your physician before starting any physical fitness program.

HEALTHY LIVING BOOKS are available for bulk purchase, special promotions, and premiums. For information on reselling and special purchase opportunities, please call us at 1-800-528-2550 and ask the the Special Sales Manager.

Cover design by Deborah Miller
Interior design by Deborah Miller and Calvin Lyte

10 9 8 7 6 5 4 3 2 1
Printed in Canada

Acknowledgments

Special thanks to my publisher Andrew Flach, my editor Andrea Au, assistant editor Alyssa Smith, photographer Peter Peck, and our models, Sean James and Don Saladino. All made working on *PowerSculpt* a pleasure. I'd also like to thank the educators in the fitness industry that have elevated the level and knowledge of fitness professionals. Special thanks to Paul Chek and Juan Carlos Santana for their inspiring workshops and seminars.

To my clients for their support and trust.

To Paul West, Director of The United States Surfing Federation, for giving me the opportunity of training team members.

Most of all to my family and friends who always believed in me.

Table of CONTENTS

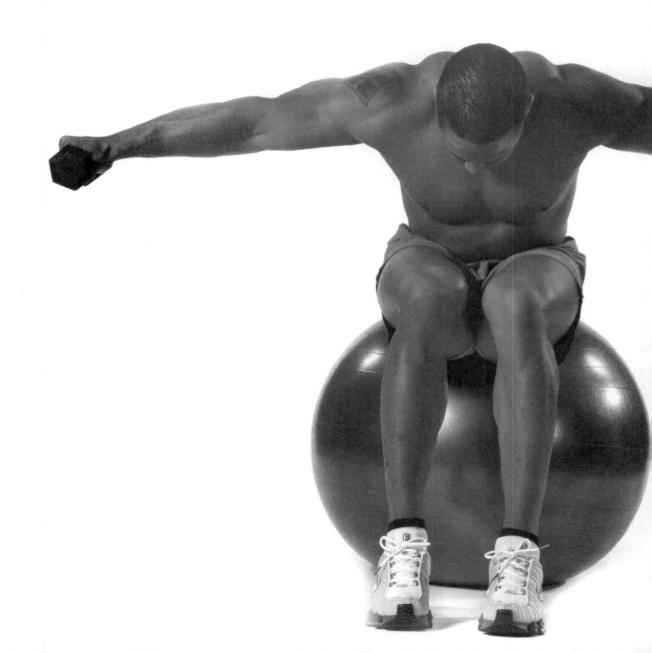

Welcome to POWER

Several years ago, an associate introduced me to the fitness ball. I struggled with every exercise she showed me. Within minutes, beads of sweat poured down my face; it felt as if I was wrestling an alligator.

I'm quite fit, so I was surprised by my inability to perform even simple exercises on the ball while maintaining my balance.

Working on the ball that day was a humbling experience, but I had a feeling that fitness ball training could open a whole new world of excellent and exciting possibilities for physical conditioning.

That first experience led me to Paul Chek and Juan Carlos Santana, two of the nation's leading fitness experts and educators, and two of the best sources of fitness ball training available. Their courses were priceless to me.

I began a daily regimen of working out on the ball. After I developed sufficient skill and knowledge, I began sharing what I had learned about the ball with my clients, some of whom achieved staggering accomplishments. Mark, an avid windsurfer, was looking to increase his conditioning so that he could more quickly advance in skill. After four months of training on a fitness ball, he had never felt stronger in the water. Fitness ball training was quickly transferred into improving his windsurfing skill.

SCULPT

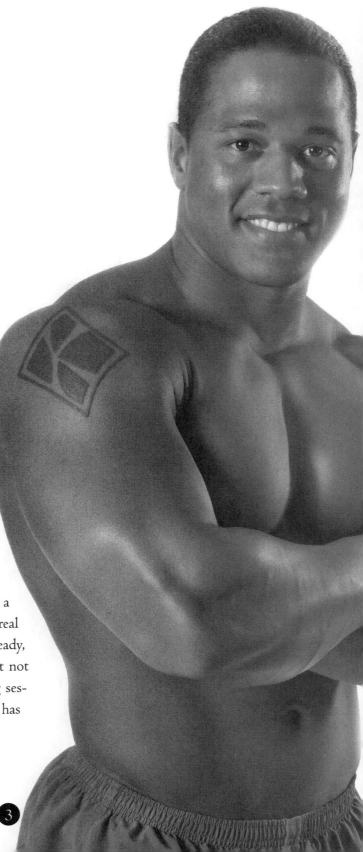

John, a 60-year-old executive, was very athletic and recently discovered a passion for golf. Unfortunately, he developed a slight herniated disk in his lower back. The fitness ball regimen I created for John strengthened his core musculature, stabilizing his lower back, reducing his pain, and putting him back on the course.

Jim was a super fit dive instructor. You would never know he was 54 years old. A former college wrestler, he had done it all when it came to getting fit. Jim was looking for a workout that was challenging, made him feel good, and had real results. Because Jim was quite proficient with free weights already, his training on a fitness ball took off. Of course you might not think so if you had seen him in his first couple of training sessions! But with the tenacity of a wrestler, he kept at it and has never felt so strong.

Sure, the evidence was anecdotal, but it proved even to someone as thick-headed as me the value of fitness ball training. I didn't have to wait for the scientific research to catch up to what I saw with my own eyes.

Armed with this newly found enthusiasm and a couple of dozen fitness balls, I designed a group fitness class and launched it at The Hamptons Boot Camp, a series of fitness classes I taught in Amagansett, New York, a few years back. The fitness ball class quickly became the most popular one offered. If fitness ball training received such a positive response and produced such wonderful results for the average person, I thought, how would it work for elite athletes?

I got my opportunity to find out when I was invited to travel with and train members of the United States Surfing Federation during a competition in the Dominican Republic. It was a richly rewarding experience. Working with these amazing athletes further expanded my knowledge of and experience with the ball. I challenged them to highly complex movements and they took to the training like fish to water. Surfers love exercises that stimulate and challenge their balance systems. And though they were quite proficient at many of the advanced exercises, I was surprised at how they struggled with some of the basic stretches. It was further evidence that the repetitive movements required by sports can create imbalances in the body. If those imbalances are not checked, poor postural habits and injuries can result.

It was rewarding to hear those surfers acknowledge how fitness ball training enhanced their performance in the sport they love, and I'm sure many of them will be traveling with their fitness balls in tow.

Birth of the Ball

The fitness ball—also known as the Swiss ball, physio ball, or stability ball—was invented in the mid-1960s by an Italian toy manufacturer. It was first used in physical rehabilitation by Swiss spinal rehab specialist Dr. Susan Klein-Vogelbach, who used the ball to help patients with orthopedic and other medical problems.

Connecting with Your Core

Core is a popular buzzword in fitness training these days. But what exactly is the core and why is it so important? Like the steel cables of a bridge, your core is the foundation and support system of your body. It stabilizes your spine and connects your upper and lower extremities. It is the central source of power and is essential for efficient movement. Furthermore, your core is your center of gravity, playing an essential role in helping you maintain balance and equilibrium. In short, a strong and stable core is crucial to optimum health and movement—whether you're hanging ten on your surfboard or carrying your groceries from the store and stepping off the curb.

Technically speaking, the core musculature includes your spine, your pelvic and shoulder girdles, and the muscles that act on these bony structures (back and hip muscles).

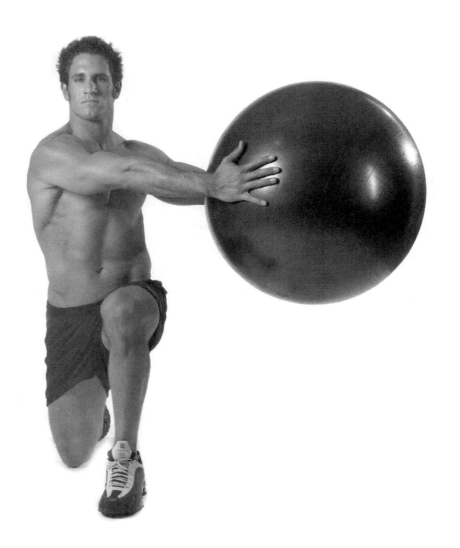

The Ball Today

These days, fitness ball training is being integrated with yoga, Pilates, pre- and postnatal exercise, senior exercise regimens, everyday flexibility, and functional training.

Working on the fitness ball not only helps develop the strength of your core muscles, but, because the ball is unstable, training on it also strengthens your stabilizing muscles. Those muscles are found at major joints and around your spine, hips, and shoulders. Most people don't train their stabilizing muscles, concentrating instead on the so-called major muscle groups of the chest, back, shoulders, hamstrings, quadriceps, biceps, and triceps. For those muscle groups to work together, create explosive movements, and lessen the possibility of injury, the smaller stabilizing muscles must be trained and well conditioned, too. Training on the ball also strengthens your joints, and

Change is Good

If you never change your exercise routines, you'll never change your body. That's because over time your body adapts to the same routine. If you want to become stronger and more fit, then you must constantly change your workouts. Changing the speed, intensity, and stability of an exercise will do just that. And the fitness ball is the only piece of equipment that will allow you to do that.

strong joints allow your body to move more powerfully, with more fluidity, and with less chance of injury.

The PowerSculpt Difference

Tired of the same old exercise routine: ten reps, wait, and do it again; waiting in line at the gym to use the new machine—that turns out to be as useless as the old machine?

If you're looking for a workout that will charge you up, give you fast results, is stimulating and fun, then look no further, because I promise you that PowerSculpt is like no other you've ever experienced.

Regardless of how old you are, what condition you're in, or what kinds of training you're accustomed to, the PowerSculpt Workout will get you to the next level, safely and progressively. It's not an easy workout; even a well-conditioned athlete will most likely need to start at the beginning levels, so don't get down on yourself if you tire quickly. Those twenty to thirty minutes of training per session for the first two to three weeks will be challenging. Why? Because of the way the ball stimulates your central nervous system and the synergistic kinesiology of fitness ball training. In other words, when you do the PowerSculpt Workout, you're bringing all your muscles to the party. You may be doing a chest exercise, but at the same time you'll be working your lower back, hips, butt, and legs. Or you might be focusing on an abdominal exercise and at the same time be working your chest, shoulders, and hip flexors. And if that's not enough, you will simultaneously be required to maintain your balance and posture.

You see, the PowerSculpt Workout doesn't isolate muscles the way those big clunky machines at the gym do. Muscle isolation is fine if you're a body builder, but most of the rest of us want a body that's lean, flexible, able to react quickly and fluidly, and works as a whole unit. Let's say you have to push a really heavy shopping cart, for example. It's not just your chest muscles that are doing the work. Your chest will work with your back, abs, legs, and myriad other muscles to create the power and movement you need. At the same time you need to maintain your balance to get proper leverage. There are no machines in the gym that will teach you how to do that. PowerSculpt does.

PowerSculpt will develop your strength through stability and balance. Your posture will change, you will become more poised, your flexibility will increase, and you'll lose inches, because of greater caloric burn resulting from the recruitment of more muscles. As your strength and balance increase, so will your level of training. You'll be able to chart your progress and execute movements you never thought possible. After awhile, what you once considered a workout will be a warm-up. If you're looking to burn fat and tone your body, PowerSculpt is the road map that will get you there.

About the PowerSculpt Workouts

In the pages that follow, you'll learn everything you need to know about working out with the fitness ball. You'll start with balance and stability exercises, which are important because they help you identify your starting level.

After that you'll move on to the PowerSculpt 10-Minute Warm-Up. Do those exercises in sequence as a prelude to the more challenging workouts to come.

Chapter 4 is where you'll learn all the PowerSculpt moves. These exercises will challenge your stability, work your core, and strengthen and sculpt your whole body. They are also the exercises you'll use for the PowerSculpt Workouts.

In chapters 5 and 6, I acquaint you with some moves and poses designed especially to enhance your flexibility and balance.

Chapter 7 is where it all comes together in the PowerSculpt Workout, a progressive 12-week body sculpting plan. It couldn't be simpler: One hour a day, two or three days a week for 12 weeks. But I don't just throw you on the ball and wish you luck. My workouts guide you from the very beginning (Phase 1: Foundation and Adaptation) to an advanced body sculpting workout (Phase 3: Power and Performance).

I saved the best workout for last. It's the PowerSculpt Body Blast Circuit Workout. It's just one body part per day—12 to 15 minutes—for five days a week.

So again, welcome to PowerSculpt. With the ball and this book, I guarantee you a workout like you've never experienced!

Chapter 1

The Power of PROPER POSTURE

Good posture is essential for good balance and energy. Almost every popular form of exercise—Feldenkrais®, Pilates, yoga—is based on achieving proper posture. In fact, Dr. Feldenkrais said, "Posture is where movement begins and ends."

Where would you prefer to stand if you were to swing a bat, club, or racket? How about throwing a punch, tossing a football, kicking, or high jumping? Would you rather be on a rowboat or a battleship? Your performance is as good as your stability and your stability is most optimal when you have good posture. Think posture is for sissies? Tell that to the NFL players or the top rugby players who take ballet and yoga to improve posture, power, and performance.

Posture is nothing new. We have as a sedentary society developed poor postural habits. Observe photos of Native Americans, Africans, and aboriginal tribes. Do you ever notice them with poor posture? Of course not. When you spend the days hunting, fishing, running, and doing all the chores necessary to survive, your body becomes strong

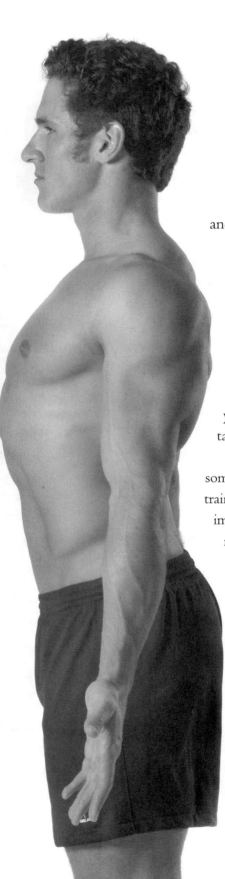

and posturally correct out of necessity.

We must be aware of our posture every day, not only when we exercise. But what is good posture? Chances are your posture isn't perfect. Tightness in one set of muscles and weakness in others can certainly affect your ability to stand up straight. Playing sports that require repetitive movements and performing small tasks in your everyday life can have adverse effects on your posture. When you sit at your desk do you cross your legs? When standing, do you always lean on your dominant leg? Do you carry a pack over one shoulder? Poor habits created over years take constant positive reeducation.

If you begin PowerSculpt with poor posture (we all have it to some degree) you need to pay close attention to your form while training. The good news is that awareness is the first step toward improvement and PowerSculpt will strengthen and stretch the muscles needed for better posture. Some of my clients have achieved positive postural changes in a matter of months. Funny thing is, they were constantly being told how wonderful they looked and asked how much weight they had lost, when all they really did was improve their posture.

Proper Posture for PowerSculpt

How important is posture when it comes to PowerSculpt? Well, it governs whether or not you will be able to progress to more advanced exercises and avoid injury. If you try to advance through the exercises too quickly, you not only risk injuring yourself, but you also reinforce poor postural movements and habits that are hard to relearn.

Here are the most important elements of proper posture:

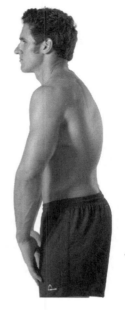

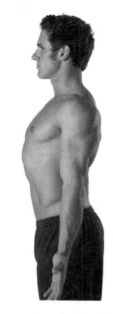

Protraction. The shoulder blades spread apart like you're hugging a tree.

Retraction. The shoulder blades are pinched together. Their optimal position when you're doing upper body exercises is retracted and depressed *(see below)*.

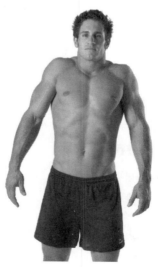

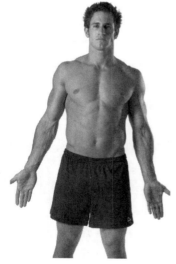

Elevation. Shoulders are up around your ears.

Depression. Shoulders are down and in a stable position.

Neck. Jutting jaw or forward placement of the head is among the most common postural issues. Using machines that support the head while you do crunches or interlacing your fingers to support the back of your head exacerbates the problem. If you have weak neck flexors and hold the back of your head to eliminate the stress, you're just keeping those muscles weak. At the same time, you're strengthening your abdominals. It all adds up to forward head placement.

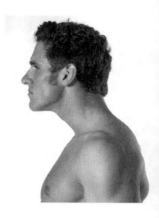

I might be crazy, but if my forearms got sore twirling my Mom's pasta with a fork, I wouldn't stop eating the pasta; I'd make my forearms stronger! If your neck needs support when you do crunches, I suggest you do what you'd do for any other weak muscles: Strengthen them. Once you've achieved good postural form, you can follow the Neck strengthening exercises that start on page 113.

Shoulders. The shoulder girdle is one of the most complex joints of the human body. Maintaining strong, stable, flexible shoulders is necessary to your well-being. But finding proper shoulder position isn't easy. In a natural, relaxed state, the shoulder blades will be in a "seated" position at the upper back. The chest will be open and wide without the points of the upper arms (shoulders) pointed forward. The tops of the shoulders should also be depressed, creating a large space between them and your ears. Your shoulders have four primary positions: depression, elevation, protraction, and retraction.

Neutral Spine. Neutral spine, or neutral posture, is the proper alignment of the body between the postural extremes of posterior tilt and anterior tilt (right). In neutral spine, the body is able to function in its strongest, most balanced position and stress to the joints, muscles, and vertebrae is minimized. Finding and maintaining the neutral spine position helps you decrease the risk of injury and increase the efficiency of any exercises you do. The neutral spine position is different for everyone and finding it isn't always easy. Performing the Rotations (page 28) and Pelvic Tilts (page 29), which you'll find in the the PowerSculpt 10-Minute Warm-Up, will help you become aware of your pelvic movement, and that's the first step in finding your neutral spine.

Another way to find your neutral posture is to lie on your back on the floor. Bend your knees and place your feet about hip width apart and flat on the floor. You may be tempted to press your lower back into the floor, but don't. Now, place the heels of your hands on your hip bones and then place the index finger of each hand on your pubic bone. Your hands should be forming a triangle. When you're in the neutral spine position, that triangle will be flat, parallel to the floor.

As you do the PowerSculpt Workout, keep in mind the importance of proper posture. Remember: Form is everything. Without it, not only are the exercises less effective, but they may in fact do harm.

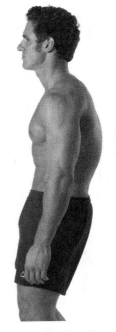

Posterior Tilt. Shoulders are rounded forward, the neck juts forward, and the butt sags.

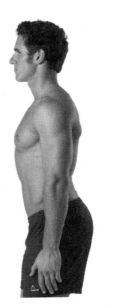

Anterior Tilt. Tight hip flexors pull your hips forward; your butt is out, and your lower back is curved inward.

PowerSculpt Tips

• When you exercise on the fitness ball, remember to **tuck your belly button into your spine.** A tight belly engages the **transverse abdominis,** the deepest of the abdominal muscles and the major stabilizer of the lower back.

• ***Pain should never be part of exercise.*** If you do experience pain while exercising, stop. Perhaps your posture needs to be reassessed or maybe you're trying to progress too quickly.

Chapter 2

Getting ACQUAINTED with the FITNESS BALL

PowerSculpt is for you, no matter what your level of fitness. However, getting used to working on the fitness ball can be tricky because it's a ball and, well, balls are not stable—they tend to roll. It will take time to awaken your body's stabilizing muscles; but as your brain adapts to the stimuli it receives from your nervous system in response to training on a fitness ball, you'll learn to maintain proper posture. Once you've developed and charted your ability to stabilize yourself, you can choose the PowerSculpt Workout that's right for your fitness level. From there, you can progress to more challenging workouts. Progressing in this manner is safe and effective and will ensure that your muscles work in synergy while you perform the exercises.

Fitness Ball Basics

When you shop for a fitness ball, you'll soon discover that it's not a one-size-fits-all piece of equipment. There are several sizes available. But in the world of PowerSculpt, size matters. So here's how to choose a fitness ball that's right for you: When you sit on the ball, your thighs should be parallel to the floor and your knees bent at a 90-degree angle.

Of course, this is a rule of thumb. You can use a larger or smaller ball to change the nature

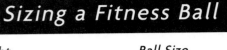

Sizing a Fitness Ball	
Height	*Ball Size*
Up to 4'10" (145 cm)	Small 18" (45 cm)
4'10" – 5'5" (145–165 cm)	Medium 22" (55 cm)
5'5" – 6'0" (165–185 cm)	Large 26" (65 cm)
6'0" – 6'5" (185–195 cm)	X-Large 30" (75 cm)

Depending on your individual needs (sitting or exercising) you may need different sizes.

of an exercise—be it a stretch or a balance or strength exercise. So once you're familiar with the workouts, experiment with different sizes—it's challenging and fun!

In addition to the ball's size, the level of inflation can change the intensity of the exercise. For PowerSculpt, I recommend keeping the ball firmly inflated, but always follow the manufacturer's directions.

Balance and Stability on the Ball

So you know which ball is right for you; now all that's left is hopping on, right? Well, not quite. Remember, this is a ball we're talking about, and when you try to simply "hop" on, it's likely to roll around a bit. That can be either annoying, unnerving, or even scary, depending on your temperament.

But don't give up. All it takes is a little time and the exercises on the following pages.

Those exercises are broken out into two sets: The first three exercises will help you get onto the ball and balance with confidence. The second set of exercises allows you to gauge your stability on the ball. That's important, because knowing your level of stability lets you choose the PowerSculpt Workout that's right for you. So as you do the Stability Test moves, keep track of your progress.

GETTING
Onto the BALL

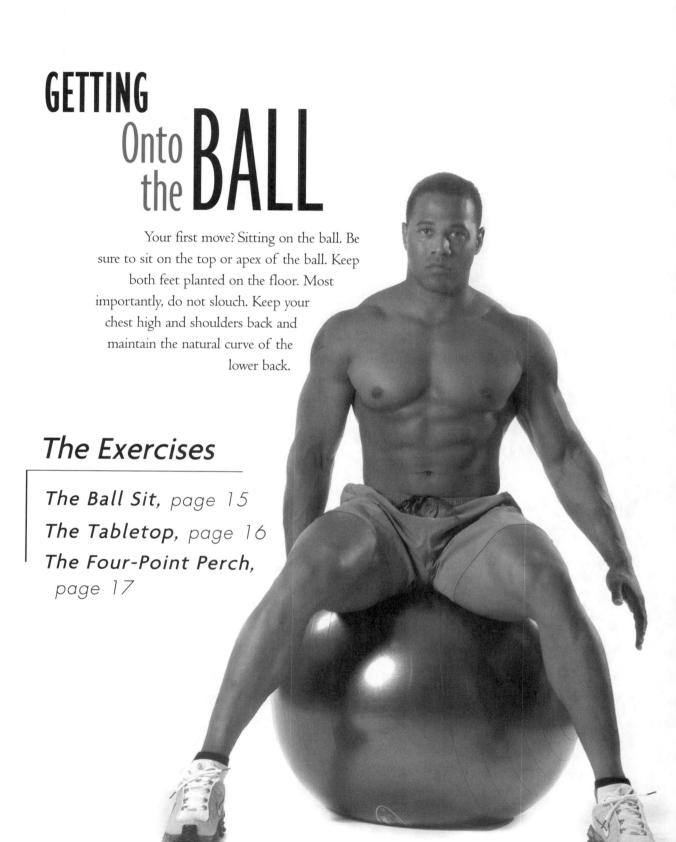

Your first move? Sitting on the ball. Be sure to sit on the top or apex of the ball. Keep both feet planted on the floor. Most importantly, do not slouch. Keep your chest high and shoulders back and maintain the natural curve of the lower back.

The Exercises

The Ball Sit, page 15
The Tabletop, page 16
The Four-Point Perch, page 17

The Ball Sit

TECHNIQUE & FORM
Place the ball next to a wall. Sit on the apex of the ball with your feet shoulder width apart. Your ears, shoulders, and hips should be in alignment. Once you feel confident, move the ball away from the wall.

If this is your introduction to the fitness ball, you will be surprised at how enjoyable just sitting on the ball can be. Use it as a chair at the office or at home. It will encourage good posture and engage and strengthen your core musculature.

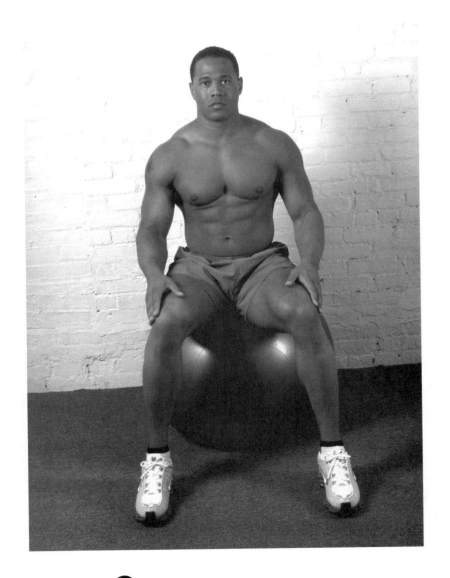

The Tabletop

The Tabletop position is an important part of a variety of chest and hip exercises. The position will strengthen the hips, glutes, hamstrings, and lower back.

TECHNIQUE & FORM

Sit on the apex of the ball with your feet shoulder width apart. Slowly walk your feet forward, letting the ball roll slowly up your back to your shoulders. Stop and elevate your hips so that they're parallel to the floor. Your head and neck should be resting comfortably on the ball and your feet flat on the floor.

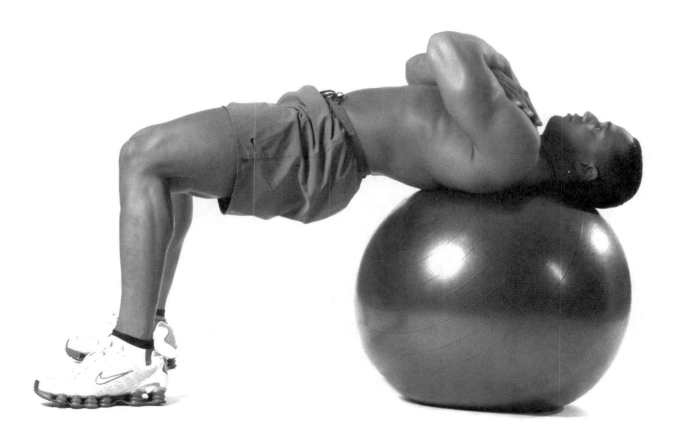

Four-Point Perch

The **Four-Point Perch** is the initial phase of an advanced balance position. Becoming confident and efficient in the **Four-Point Perch** is essential before attempting advanced balance positions.

Paul's Pro Tip
If you find the **Four-Point Perch** difficult, begin with your knees on the ball and both hands on the floor. Alternate taking each hand off the floor and placing it on the ball until you're able to take both hands off the floor.

TECHNIQUE & FORM

Stand in front of the ball with your feet shoulder width apart. Gently place your knees against the ball and both hands on top of the ball. Roll forward so that your feet come off of the ground; balance in this position for as long as you feel comfortable).

VARIATION

Perching with your hands on the floor is the beginning position for The Perch. Begin with your hands on the floor and your knees on the ball. This should feel relatively stable. As your stability increases, take one hand off the floor and touch the ball. Alternate hands.

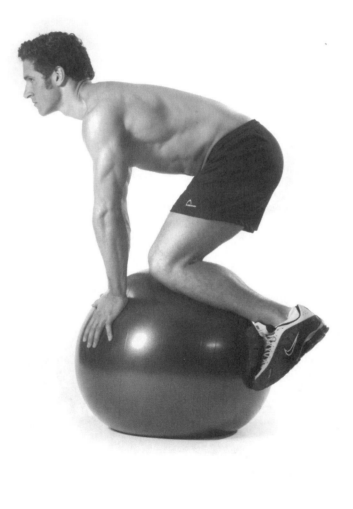

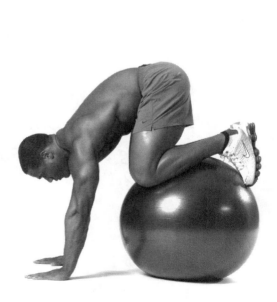

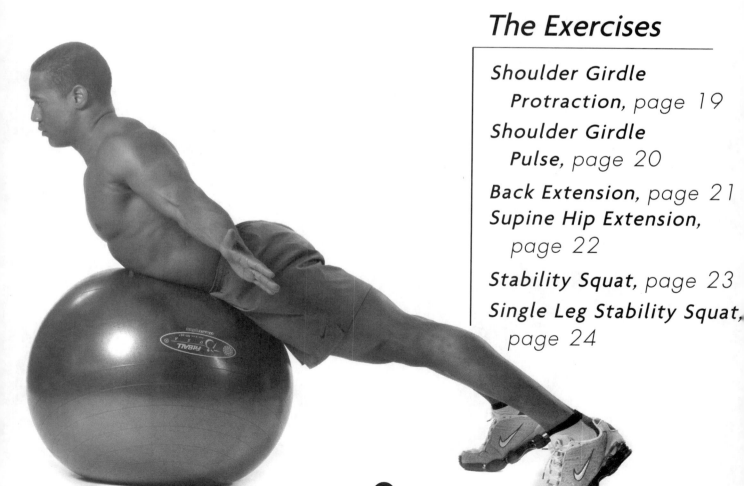

PowerSculpt
STABILITY Tests

These moves will help you choose the
PowerSculpt Workout level that's right
for you, so be sure to keep track
of how long you can hold each
of these poses.

The Exercises

Shoulder Girdle Protraction

The *Shoulder Girdle Protraction* lets you know how strong your shoulder girdle is— and that's important information to have before you try any high-intensity upper-body exercises.

TECHNIQUE & FORM

Place your knees on the ball and your hands on the floor as though you were about to do a push-up. Don't allow your hips to dip; keep your head aligned with your spine. Spread your shoulder blades as far apart as possible.

Beginner: Hold the position for 20 seconds.

Advanced: Hold the position for more than 60 seconds.

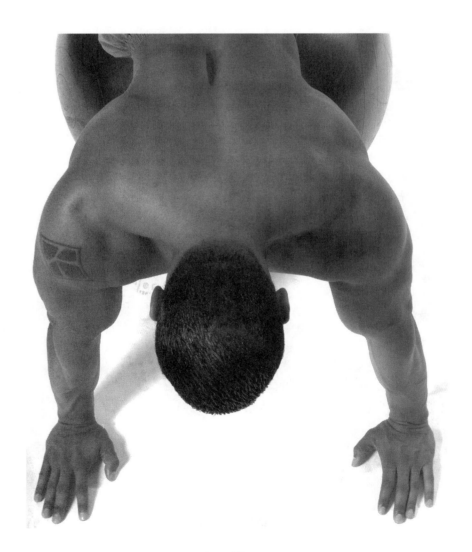

Shoulder Girdle Pulse

The *Shoulder Girdle Pulse* is an excellent exercise for strengthening the serratis anterior, which is a major stabilizer of the shoulder scapulas.

TECHNIQUE & FORM

Place your knees on the ball and your hands on the floor as though you were about to do a push-up. Don't allow your hips to dip; keep your head aligned with your spine. Spread your shoulder blades as far apart as possible and then squeeze them together again.

Beginner: Do 3 sets of 10.

Advanced: Do 3 sets of 15.

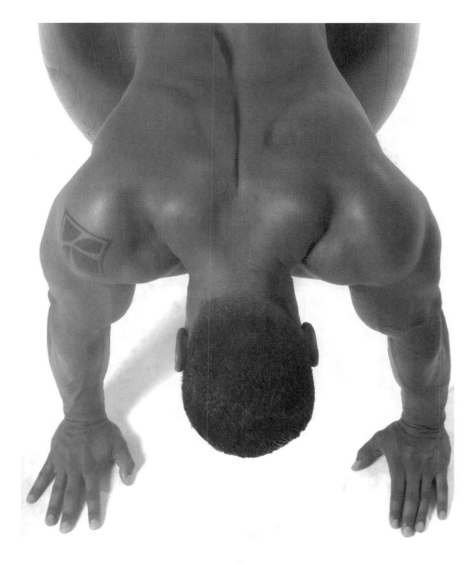

Back Extension

When performed on a fitness ball, the *Back Extension* will strengthen the para-spinal muscles. These deep back muscles are critical to have a healthy back.

TECHNIQUE & FORM

Place the front of your hips on the ball; extend your legs behind you with your feet wide apart and your toes on the floor. Place your arms next to your sides. Lift your chest off of the ball and rotate your hands toward floor. Squeeze your shoulder blades together.

Beginner: Hold the position for 30 seconds

Advanced: Hold the position for 3 minutes.

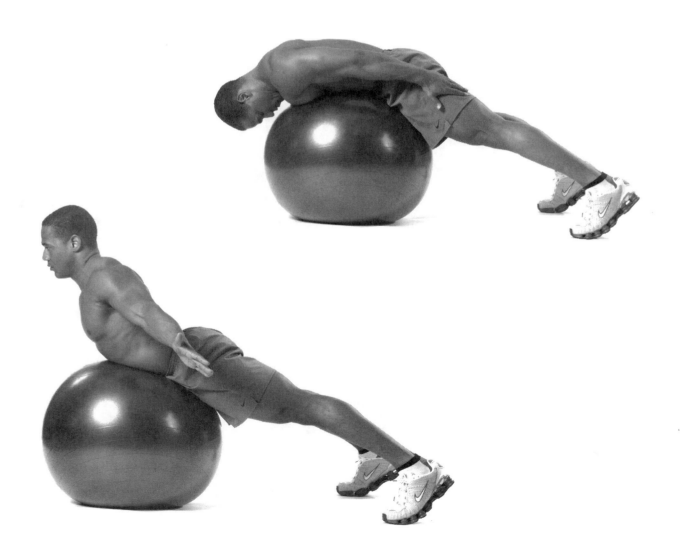

Supine Hip Extension

The *Supine Hip Extension* will increase the strength of the extensor chain and encourage the lower back, butt, and hamstrings to work in synergy.

TECHNIQUE & FORM

Lie on your back on the floor; place your ankles on top of the ball. Spread your arms out to your sides with your palms up. Elevate your hips so that your ankles, hips, and shoulders are in a straight line.

Beginner: Hold the position for 30 seconds.

Advanced: Hold the position for 3 minutes.

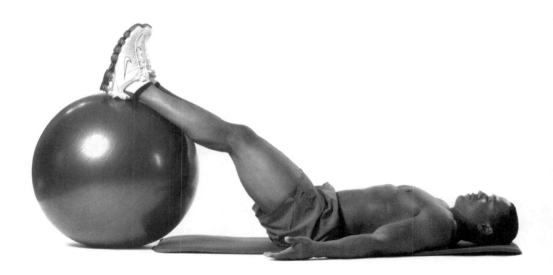

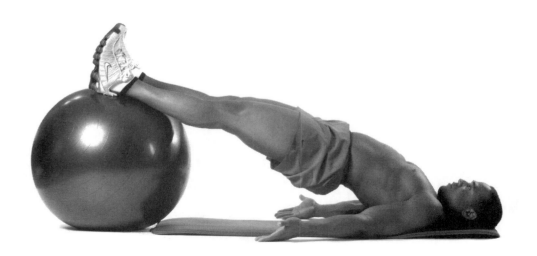

Stability Squat

The *Stability Squat* is the king of lower body exercises. In this version you won't raise and lower yourself. Instead, see how long you can hold the down position to gauge your stability.

Paul's Pro Tip
Keep focused on long, deep breaths and keep your face, shoulders, and hands relaxed.

TECHNIQUE & FORM
Stand about two feet from a wall. Place the ball between your lower back and the wall. Lower yourself until your thighs are parallel to floor. Hold yourself in the down position. DO NOT place your hands on top of your thighs; let them hang by your side. Your knees should be in line with your first two toes. do not let your knees come over the plane of the toes.

Beginner: Hold position for 30 seconds.
Advanced: Hold position for 3 minutes.

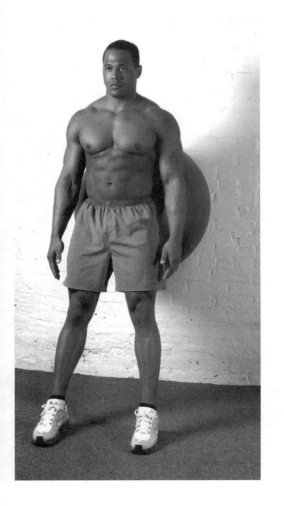

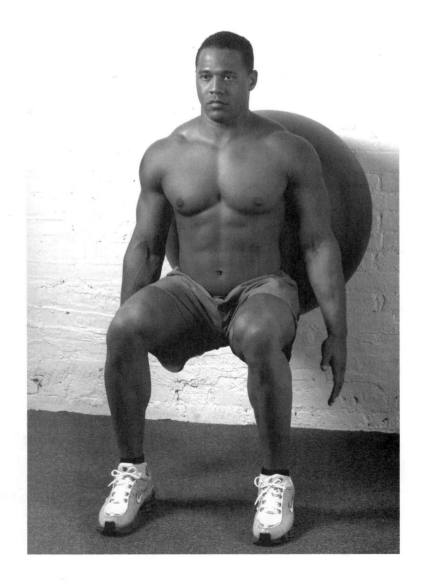

Single-Leg Stability Squat

Once you've mastered the Stability Squat on the previous page, move on to this one, which further challenges the stability of the ankles, knees, and hips.

Paul's Pro Tip
Don't place your hands on your thighs; let them hang by your side or hold them parallel to the floor.

TECHNIQUE & FORM
Stand about two feet from a wall. Place the ball between your lower back and the wall. Lift and bend one leg at a 90-degree angle. Lower yourself until your thighs are parallel to floor and hold the position. DO NOT place your hands on top of your thighs; let them hang by your side.

Beginner: Hold position for 15 seconds.

Advanced: Hold position for 1 minute, 30 seconds.

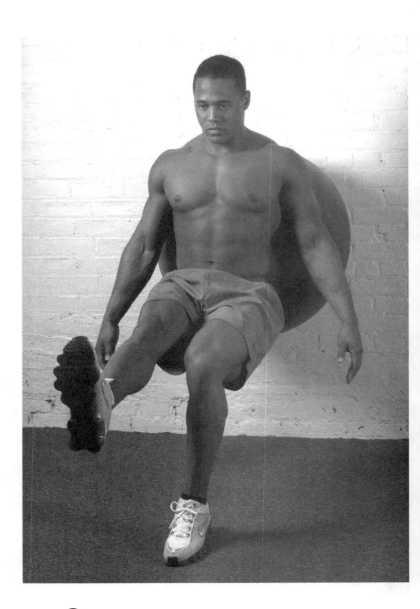

Chapter 3

The POWERSCULPT 10-Minute WARM-UP

Just as with any other exercise program, warming up before the PowerSculpt Workout is essential. An effective warm-up increases your heart rate and the blood flow to your muscles. That in turn increases your body temperature, which warms up your joints and enhances the elasticity of connective tissues, tendons, ligaments, and cartilage. Any good warm-up increases your oxygen intake, delivering nutrients to muscles and synovial fluid to joints, which lubricates them. It will also engage the neuromuscular (balance) system, charging up reaction time and coordination.

Perform these exercises in the order they're presented for a total-body warm-up. When you're finished, you'll be ready for your PowerSculpt Workout—or any other workout, for that matter!

If you're just starting out, warming up can be a workout. Keep that in mind as you work through the exercises on the next few pages. Move through as full a range of motion as you feel comfortable with. Each exercise can—and should—be modified to fit your fitness level. Remember: Pain should never be part of your exercise program.

Oh, and one last thing—have fun!

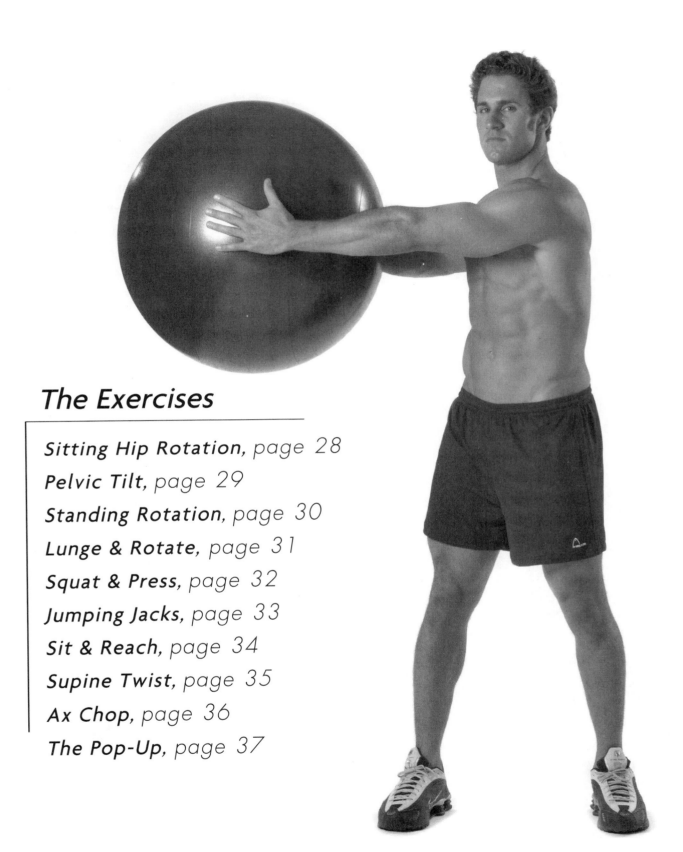

The Exercises

Sitting Hip Rotation

The *Sitting Hip Rotation* is effective on several levels: It warms up and stretches your lumbar spine and engages your sense of balance. It enhances awareness of your pelvic movements, helping you to discover your neutral spine.

Paul's Pro Tip
Keep your ears, shoulders, and hips in alignment and your shoulders and chest still throughout the exercise.

TECHNIQUE & FORM
Sit on the apex of the ball with your feet shoulder width apart. Let your hands and arms hang by your side. Make small circles with your hips. Do several in each direction.

VARIATION
Instead of making circles with your hips, do figure eights.

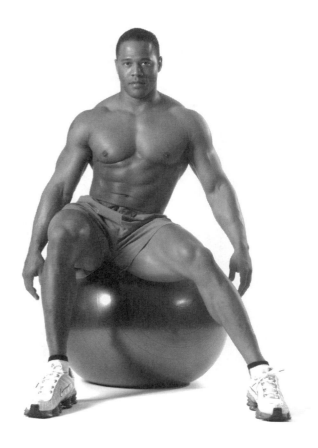
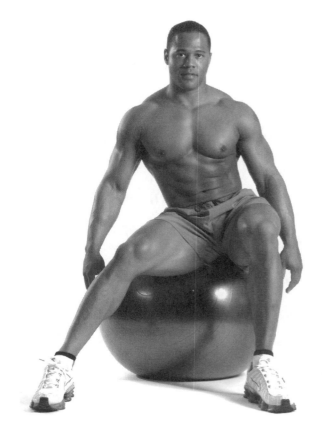

Pelvic Tilt

The **Pelvic Tilt** is one of the simplest and most effective warm-up and stretch for the lower back (lumbar spine).

Paul's Pro Tip

Avoid rocking your upper body back and forth. Keep your chest high and still. Draw the pelvis toward your chest then away from it.

TECHNIQUE & FORM

Sit on the apex of the ball with your feet shoulder width apart. Put your hands out to your sides. Gently rock your pelvis forward and backward. (You might find you have a limited range of movement. That's okay; moving as little as 1 inch is beneficial.) Your ears, shoulders, and hips should be directly in line.

VARIATIONS

Variation I: Perform the same exercise with your feet together, then again lifting one foot off the floor.

Variation II: Do this exercise with your eyes closed to challenge your sense of balance.

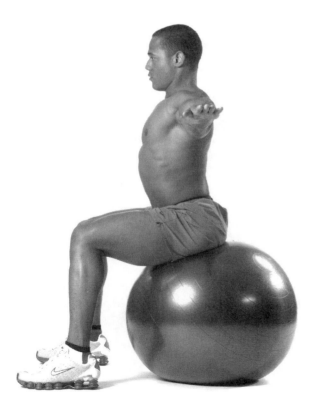
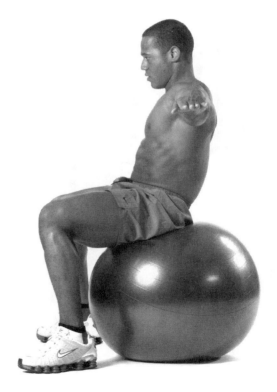

Standing Rotation

The **Standing Rotation** is an excellent warm-up for the shoulders, waist, and hips. As you get accustomed to the movements, you'll be able to increase your range of motion.

Paul's Pro Tip
Draw your belly button toward your spine and keep your abdominals tight throughout this exercise.

TECHNIQUE & FORM
Stand with your feet shoulder width apart and your knees slightly bent. Keep your belly pulled in tightly and your shoulders in their seated position. Hold the ball in your hands with your arms extended. Slowly rotate the ball in a horizontal line from right to left. Don't turn your head; keep your eyes forward.

VARIATION
As you rotate to the right, pivot your left foot. When you rotate to the left, pivot your right foot.

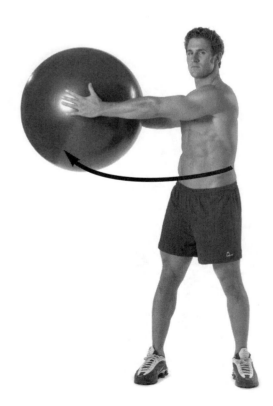
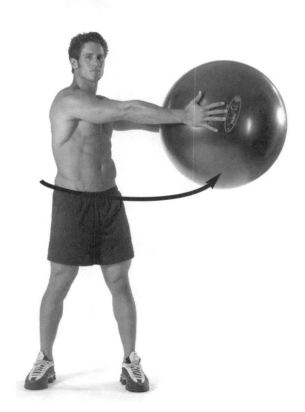

30

Lunge & Rotate

The **Lunge & Rotate** is a great full-body warm-up. It stimulates your balance and strengthens your core musculature, which stabilizes movement in your legs, hips, and shoulders.

Paul's Pro Tip

Your focus should be on the forward-moving leg, first as you decelerate your body weight, then as it pushes off the floor to return to the starting position. Be sure not to bang your rear knee on the floor.

TECHNIQUE & FORM

Stand with your feet together and your belly held in tightly. Hold the ball at chest height. Step forward and into a lunge with the right foot. As you do, rotate the ball over your left leg. Step back to the starting position and then lunge forward with the right leg, rotating the ball over the kneeling leg. Alternate for the desired number of reps.

VARIATION

Hold the ball overhead, and swing it down diagonally over the lunging leg.

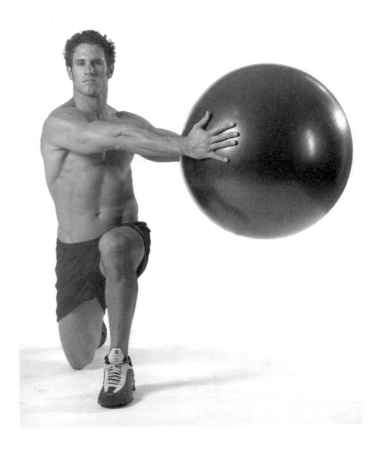

Squat & Press

The *Squat & Press* will warm you up from head to toe.

Paul's Pro Tip

Squat only as far as you can while maintaining the curve of your lower back. Be sure your feet stay firmly on the floor. If this is difficult, widen your stance and point your toes outward slightly. Those changes can help you balance and increase your range of motion.

TECHNIQUE & FORM

Stand with your chest high, your shoulders back, and your feet slightly wider than shoulder width apart. Keep your heels firmly on the ground. Hold the ball in front of you at chest level. Slowly bend your knees and lower yourself, pushing your butt back as though you're about to sit in a chair. Slowly raise yourself again, pressing the ball up over your head.

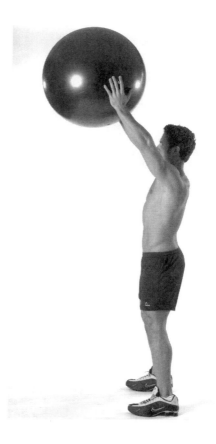
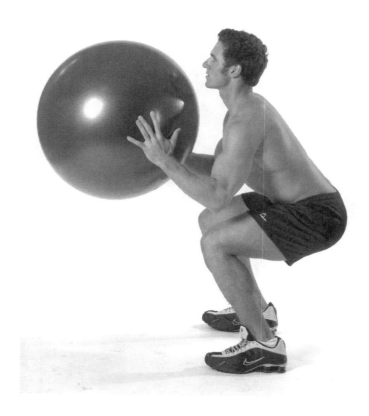

Jumping Jacks

Jumping Jacks are a fun warm-up. They'll quickly elevate your heart rate and challenge your balance and coordination.

Paul's Pro Tip

If you're having trouble balancing, keep one hand on the ball. Also, keep your back straight and avoid slouching forward.

TECHNIQUE & FORM

Sit on the apex of the ball with your feet wider than shoulder width apart. Lift your butt off the ball and drop down on it again. As you bounce, swing your arms overhead and extend your feet, raising them off the floor.

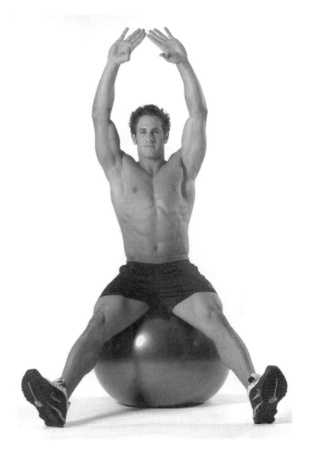 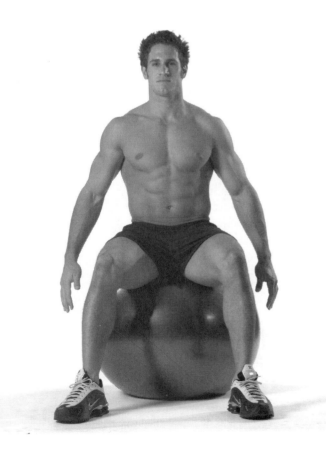

Sit & Reach

Sit & Reach will give you a full body warm-up and is an excellent stretch and warm-up for the waist, lower body, and hamstrings.

Paul's Pro Tip

Become creative with both your arm and leg positions. Try reaching your arm across your chest, or lifting one foot off of the floor as you stand.

TECHNIQUE & FORM

Sit on the apex of the ball, your feet hip distance or wider apart. Extend your arms out parallel to your shoulders. Reach one hand and touch the opposing toe. Come back to the starting position and repeat with the other side.

VARIATIONS

Variation I: You can stretch your inner thighs and groin by placing your feet even wider apart.

Variation II: Sit on the apex of the ball. Place your hands on the ball next to your hips. Stand up, keeping one hand on the ball and reaching the other in the opposite direction. Come back to the sitting position and repeat with the other side.

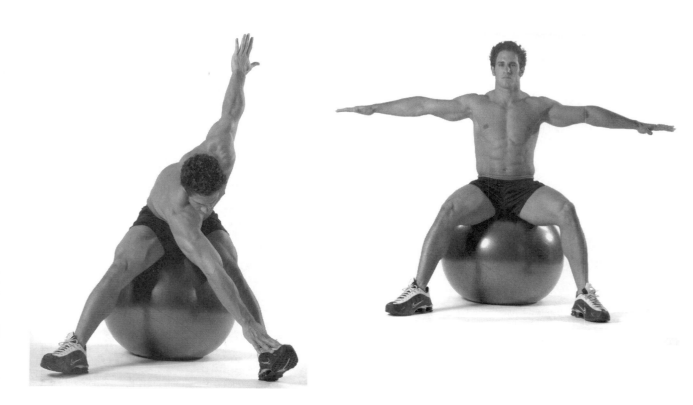

Supine Twist

TECHNIQUE & FORM

Lay face up on the floor with your arms out to the sides. Place your calves on the ball. Slowly rotate the ball in a small arc from left to right. Keep your shoulders on the floor. As you increase the range of rotation, gently rotate your head in the opposite direction of your knees.

The *Supine Twist* is a must warm-up and excellent cool-down exercise. It will help keep your spine flexible. In yoga there is a saying: "You're only as young as your spine is flexible!"

Paul's Pro Tip

Do not force an increase of your range of motion. Allow your breath and gravity to naturally increase the range of motion.

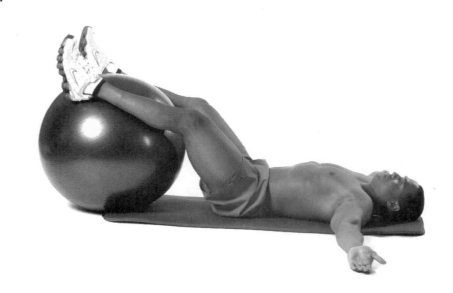

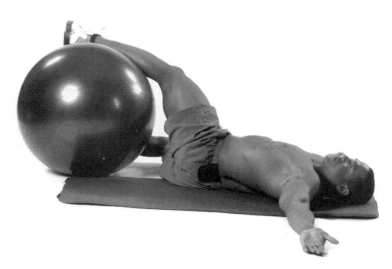

Ax Chop

The **Ax Chop** is one of the best full-body warm-up exercises. They'll get your whole body ready for rotational movements.

Paul's Pro Tip
Draw your belly into your spine to protect yor back.

TECHNIQUE & FORM
Stand with your feet shoulder width apart and your knees slightly bent. Hold the ball over your left shoulder and then swing it diagonally to the outside of your right knee. The movement should be fast. In the finish position you'll be in a half squat with your thighs parallel to the floor. Repeat on the other side.

VARIATIONS
Variation I: Reverse the movement, making an upward diagonal sweep.

Variation II: Accelerate the movement while making the upward sweep.

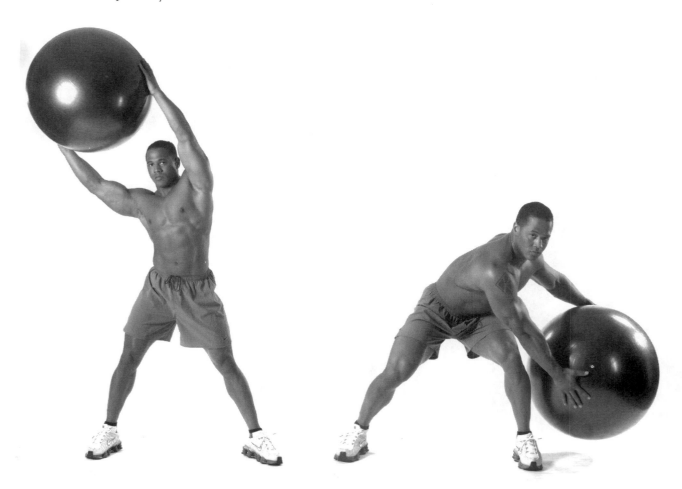

The Pop-Up

The Pop-Up is an advanced exercise which id excellent for anyone playing contact sports. If you have any sort of back problems, you should not attempt it.

Paul's Pro Tip
Use the bounce off the ball to get a good explosive lift.

TECHNIQUE & FORM

Position yourself so that your toes are on the floor and you are supporting yourself on the ball with outstretched arms. Your feet should be more than shoulder width apart. Don't let your body sag—maintain your alignment. Release your body weight and bounce onto the ball. As you come up, bring one foot alongside the ball. Bounce again and as you come up, bring the other foot alongside the ball.

VARIATIONS

Variation I: When you land, place just one hand on the ball and extend the opposite arm over your head.

Variation II: A novice's version of The Pop-Up can be done while standing with the ball held at chest height against a wall.

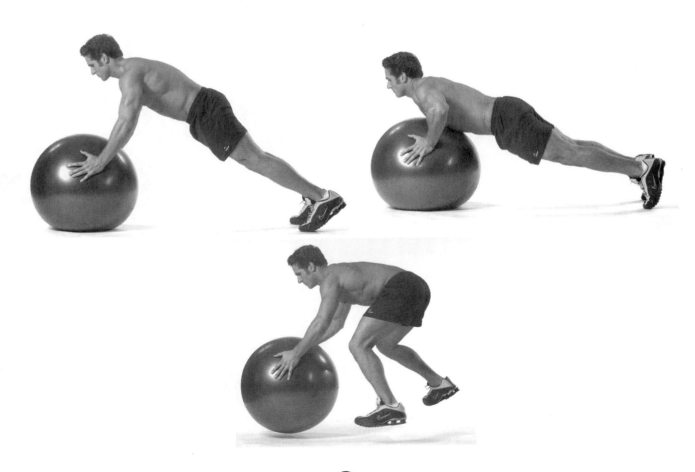

Chapter 4

The POWER

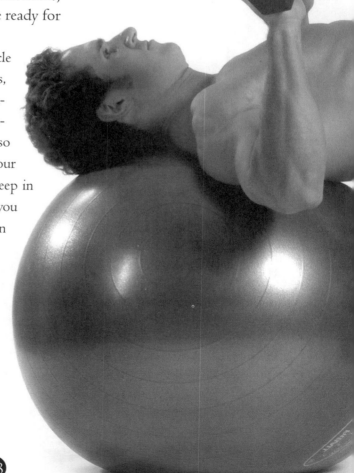

After finishing the PowerSculpt Warm-Up your heart rate should be elevated; you may have even broken a slight sweat. Now you're ready for the total-body PowerSculpt moves.

The exercises are arranged by the primary muscle groups they work: chest, back, shoulders, arms, abs, legs, glutes, and even your neck. Of course, when you're working on the fitness ball, you're never working only one muscle group. When you do chest flies, for instance, you're also challenging your sense of balance and strengthening your core. Before you start, there are some bits of advice to keep in mind. First, always stay within your range of motion. If you can't complete the exercise as described, do what you can

SCULPT
Moves

and gradually work up to the full movement. Remember that it's not unusual for even a fit individual to feel like a beginner the first couple of weeks working with the fitness ball. Second, stop immediately if you feel any pain. Third, remember the importance of proper form. Periodically take note of your posture and form on the ball and make adjustments if you need to.

Once you are familiar with all of the moves in this chapter, you'll be ready to move on to the PowerSculpt 12-Week Workouts.

PowerSculpt CHEST

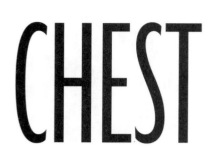

pectorals major and pectorals minor
Training your chest the PowerSculpt way will define and strengthen the chest in synergy with your core musculature. You are training in integration, not in isolation.

The Exercises

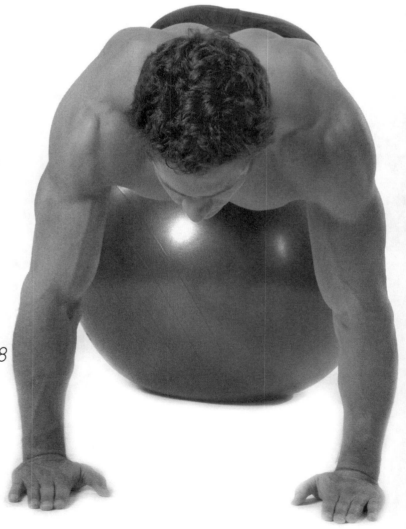

Hands-on-Floor Push-Up

When properly executed, the *Hands-on-Floor Push-Up* isn't only a chest exercise—it's also a terrific abs exercise. Doing push-ups on the ball works your core, strengthens your chest, and increases shoulder stabilization. Push-ups are among my favorite exercises because there are many variations and you can see the results so quickly.

Paul's Pro Tip
The farther away the ball is from your hips, the harder the exercise will be. It is crucial that you maintain neutral spine throughout the exercise. If your hips begin to drop, walk the ball back toward your hips to lower the intensity.

TECHNIQUE & FORM
Kneel in front of the ball, draping your hands over it. Roll out to the point of desired intensity. While in this position, (a) maintain neutral spine; (b) keep your head aligned with your spine; (c) keep your feet together on the ball; (d) keep your abs tucked in tightly (to connect the hip and shoulder). From this push-up position, lower your chest to the floor until your hands are parallel to your chest. At this point your body should be held straight. Once you can perform 10 reps without losing your form, you can progress by adding reps or increase the intensity by rolling the ball farther away from your hips.

VARIATION
As long as you maintain your alignment and form, you can let your imagination run wild. On the following pages are just a few of the most challenging push-up variations.

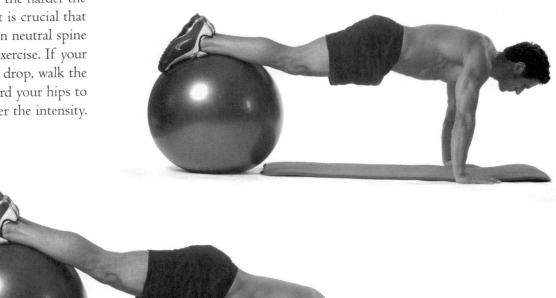

Alternating Single-Leg Push-Up

Once you've mastered the basic *Hands-on-Floor Push-Up*, challenge yourself with this version.

Paul's Pro Tip
You can avoid stress on your wrists while doing all the push-ups by keeping your fingers spread wide and distributing your weight throughout your hands and fingers.

TECHNIQUE & FORM
Kneel in front of the ball, draping your hands over it. Roll out to the point of desired intensity. Lift one leg off the ball and lower your chest to the floor until your hands are parallel to your chest. At this point your body should be held straight.

VARIATION
Extend one leg laterally to the side.

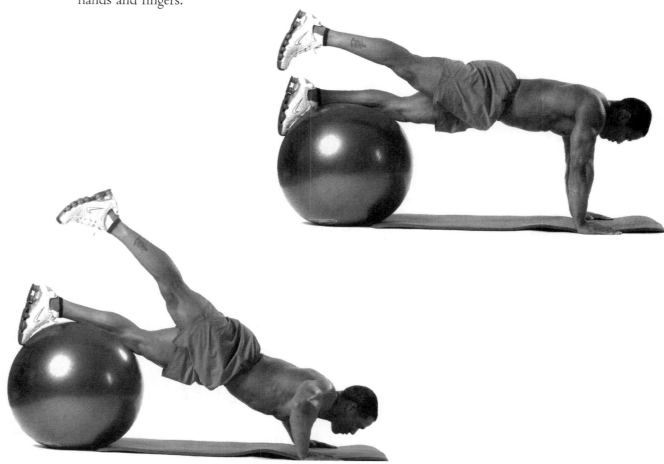

Tippy-Toe Push-Up

The *Tippy-Toe Push-Up* is the most advanced push-up you can do with both feet on the ball. Be sure to fully engage the ankle and foot muscles.

TECHNIQUE & FORM

Kneel in front of the ball, draping your hands over it. Roll out until your insteps are on the apex of the ball, and then lift yourself onto your toes. Lower your chest to the floor until your hands are parallel to your chest. At this point your body should be held straight.

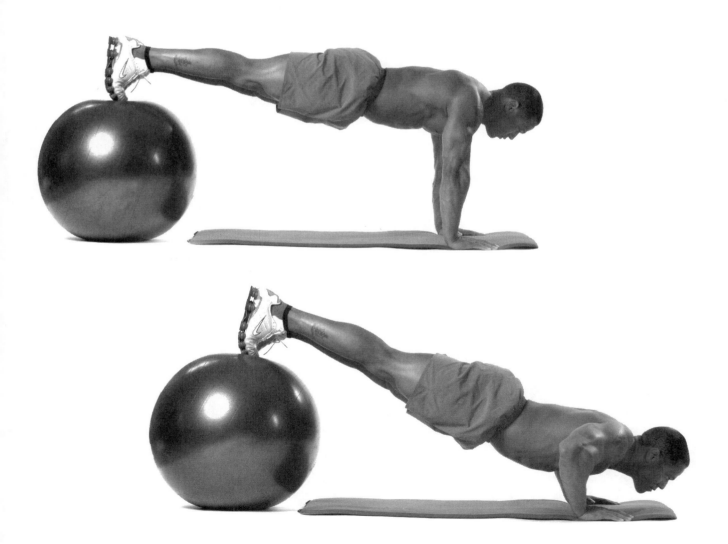

One-Legged Toe Push-Up

This advanced push-up will challenge your equilibrium, strength and balance. Be sure that you can master all the previous push-ups before attempting this exercise.

TECHNIQUE & FORM
Kneel in front of the ball, draping your hands over it. Roll out until your insteps are on the apex of the ball, and then lift yourself onto your toes. Lift one leg off of the ball and then lower your chest to the floor until your hands are parallel to your chest. At this point your body should be held straight.

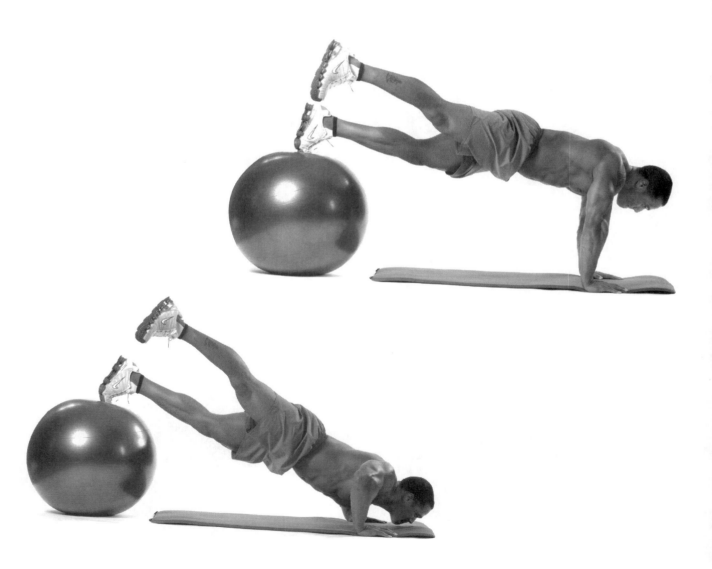

The Clapper

TECHNIQUE & FORM

Kneel in front of the ball, draping your hands over it. Roll out until your thighs are on the ball. Explode upward off the floor, clap your hands, and land on your hands again.

Master *The Clapper* and you'll impress all your friends. However, keep in mind that *The Clapper* is a very advanced polyometic exercise and should not be attempted until you have mastered the other push-ups.

Paul's Pro Tip
Start this exercise at the low intensity level by placing the ball close to your hips.

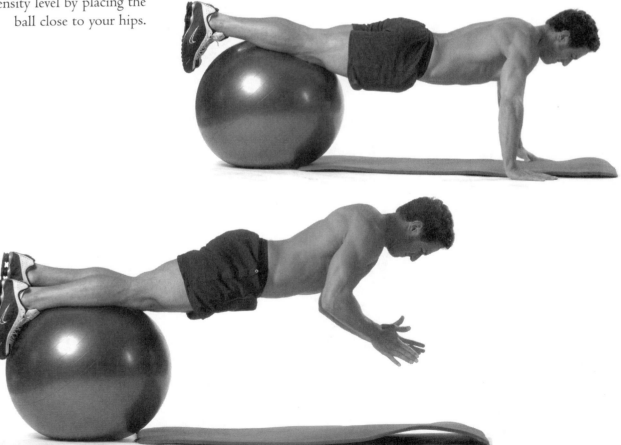

Hands-on-Ball Push-Up

As you'll discover, the *Hands-on-Ball Push-Up* is more advanced than the basic *Hands-on-Floor Push-Up*. It challenges your shoulder girdle and triceps.

Paul's Pro Tip
A good way to ease into this push-up is to start by setting the ball against a wall.

TECHNIQUE & FORM
Begin with your chest on the ball and your toes on the floor. Your feet should be wider than shoulder width apart. Place your hands on the outside of the ball with your fingers pointing toward the floor. While keeping your shoulders down and in their seated position, press your chest off of the ball, and then lower yourself again.

VARIATION
Perform the push-up with your feet together.

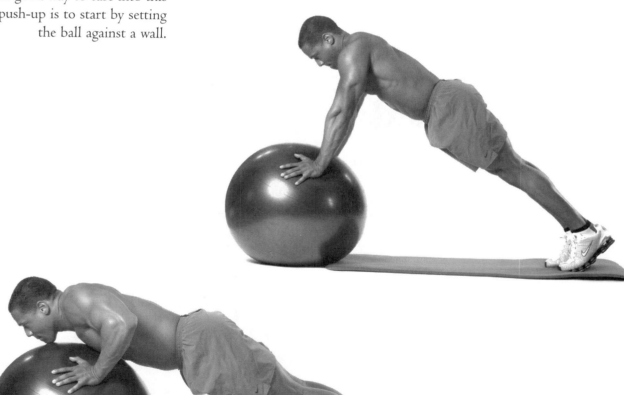

One-Legged Hands-on-Ball Push-Up

This variation of the *Hands-on-Ball Push-Up* will really test your strength and stability.

TECHNIQUE & FORM

Begin with your chest on the ball and your toes on the floor. Your feet should be shoulder width apart. Place your hands on the outside of the ball with your fingers pointing toward the floor. Lift one foot off the floor. While keeping your shoulders down and in their seated position, press your chest off of the ball, and then lower yourself again.

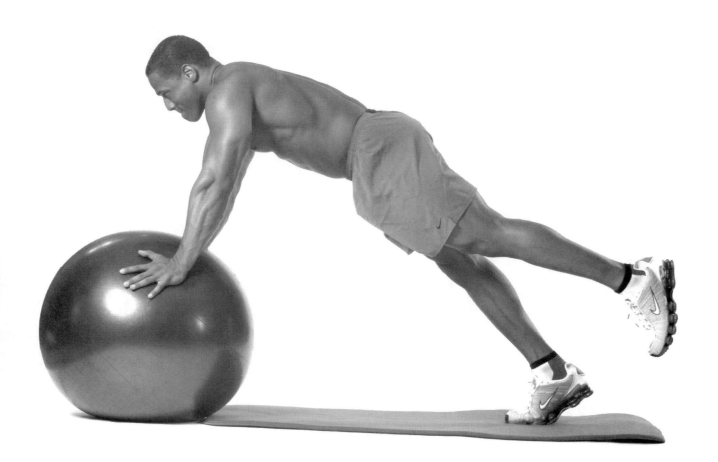

Platform Push-Up

TECHNIQUE & FORM

Kneel on a bench and place your hands on the ball so that your fingertips point to the floor. Roll the ball out to the desired intensity. (Placing more of your leg weight on the bench lessens the intensity of the exercise.) Begin with your chest on the ball and press up to the push-up.

This push-up presents a real challenge to your strength and stability. It is best to start with a wide foot stance.

Paul's Pro Tip
By changing the height of your legs, you will target different muscles in the chest and shoulders. Avoid saggy hips.

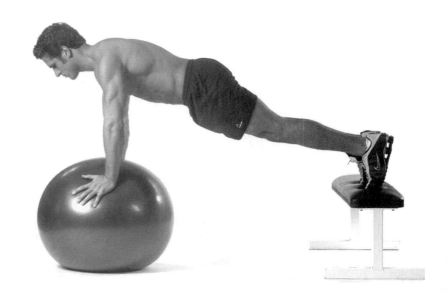

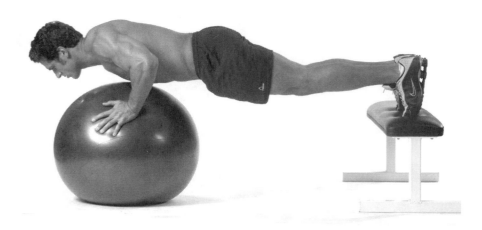

Dumbbell Flies

You can do a variety of exercises holding a weight in one or both hands. *Dumbbell Flies* sculpt and build your muscles strength, endurance, and power, depending on the results you're looking for.

Paul's Pro Tip

When the weights meet in the middle, don't let them hit each other or even click together because at that point you're no longer working your chest muscles. If your lower back aches, drop your butt slightly.

TECHNIQUE & FORM

Start with a weight you feel comfortable lifting. Sit on the apex of the ball with your feet more than shoulder width apart. Slowly walk your feet forward, letting the ball roll slowly up your back to your shoulders. Stop and elevate your hips so that they're parallel to the floor. Your head and neck should be resting comfortably on the ball and your feet should be flat on the floor. To aid your balance, move your feet even wider apart. Extend your arms up over your chest. Keeping your elbows slightly bent, open your arms until they are parallel to floor. Bring your hands back together as though you're wrapping your arms around a tree. Dumbbell flies target the center portion of the chest.

VARIATION

Try using single arm flies to seriously work your trunk and butt and challenge equilibrium. This requires strong-cross body stabilization and equilibrium. Be sure to keep your hips lifted and parallel.

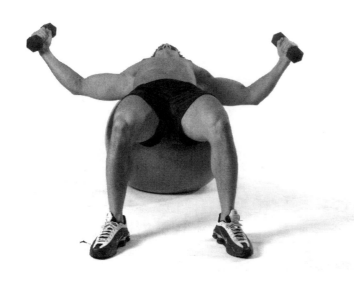
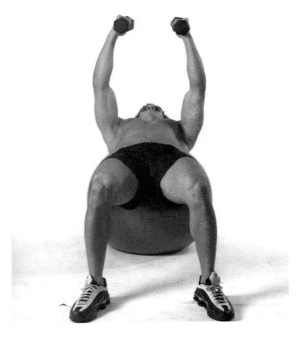

Chest Press

Doing the **Chest Press** on a fitness ball will target the chest in a more functional way than performing the exercise on a bench. It will allow for greater shoulder retraction and greater neural connection of the feet to the hands.

Paul's Pro Tip

Be sure that you keep your neck relaxed and position it on the ball so that it maintains its natural curve. Also be sure the weights stay directly over the elbows during the full range of movement.

TECHNIQUE & FORM

Start with a weight you feel comfortable with. Sit on the apex of the ball with your feet on the ground a bit wider than shoulder width apart. Hold the weights on your thighs, and slowly walk your feet forward until only your shoulders and head are resting on the ball. Lift the weights from your thigh to the starting positions—above the chest with your arms extended. Make sure your hips are elevated, keeping your knees, hips, and shoulders all in the same plane. Your knees should be directly over the ankles, with your lower and upper legs at a 90 degree angle. Lower the weight so the upper arms are parallel to your chest, then return to the starting position.

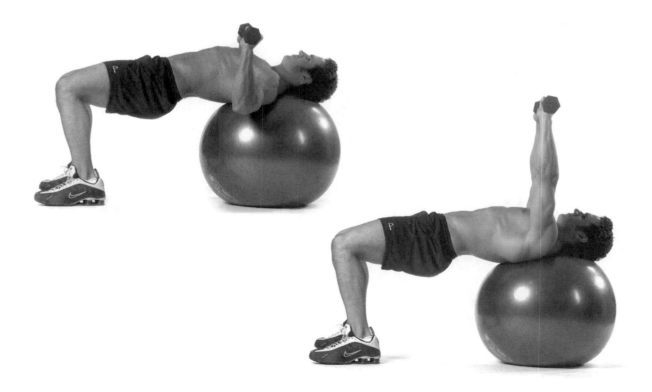

Push & Press

The **Push & Press** adds a hip extension to the usual press.

Paul's Pro Tip
The **Push & Press** engages hips, legs, and chest, resembling a full-body pressing movement.

TECHNIQUE & FORM
Start with a weight you feel comfortable lifting. Sit on the apex of the ball with your feet more than shoulder width apart. Slowly walk your feet forward, letting the ball roll slowly up your back until your head, neck, shoulders, and lower back are resting on the ball. Lower the dumbbells over your chest. As you press the dumbbells up over your chest, elevate your hips so that you're in the Tabletop position. As you lower the dumbbells, lower your hips again.

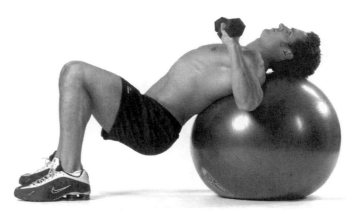

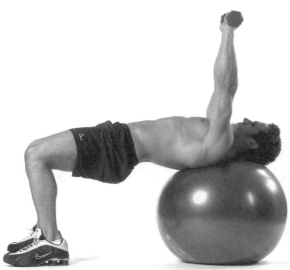

PowerSculpt

BACK

trapezius, latissimus dorsi, rhomboids, and erectors
What good is a chest that looks like a Mercedes if your back looks like a Volkswagen? A strong back is the foundation of great posture and is literally the framework from where to hang a great chest.

The Exercises

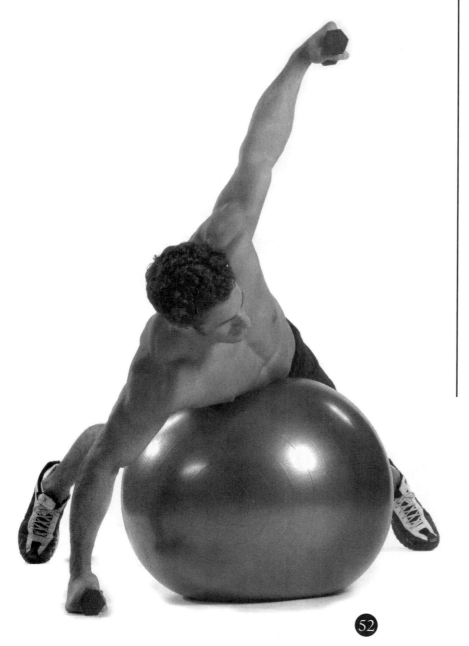

Back Extension I

TECHNIQUE & FORM
Lay with your hips on the ball and your feet wide apart behind you. Keep your knees off the floor. Place your hands, palms up, by your thighs. Lift your chest off the ball, rotate your palms toward the floor, and squeeze your shoulder blades together. Hold the up position for 3 seconds and then return to the starting position.

This stability test also strengthens your back, by holding the up position for 3 seconds.

Paul's Pro Tip
Be sure to keep your head and neck in alignment with your spine. Do not hyperextend your neck.

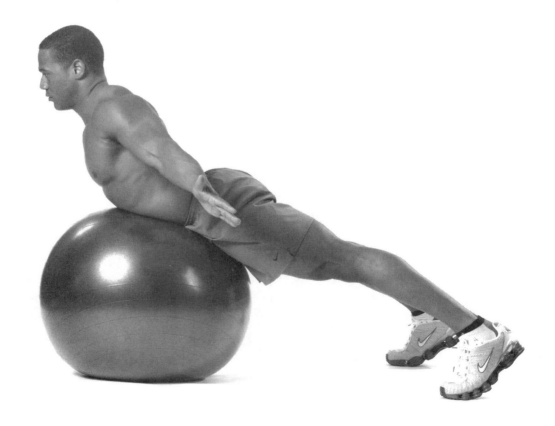

Back Extension II

The **Back Extension II** requires a bit more back strength and stability.

Paul's Pro Tip
Be sure to keep your thumbs pointed up to engage your shoulder girdle.

TECHNIQUE & FORM

Lay with your hips on the ball and your feet wide apart behind you. Keep your knees off the floor. Place your hands, palms up, by your thighs. Lift your chest off the ball. As you do, squeeze your shoulder blades together and extend your arms in front of you. Hold the up position for 3 seconds and then return to the starting position.

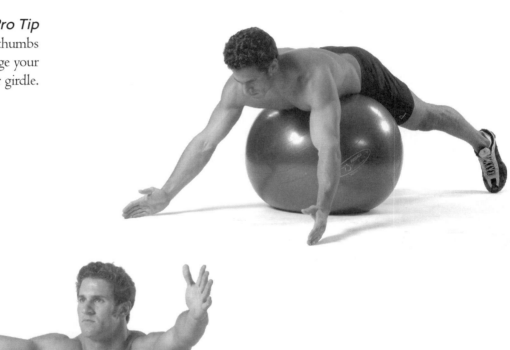

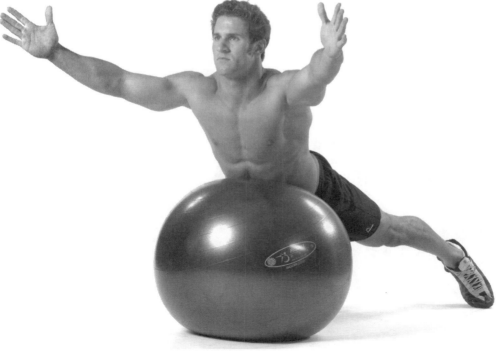

Dead Lift on Ball

Doing the **Dead Lift on Ball** puts a challenging twist to a great exercise. You will feel your thighs and buttocks burning. Always maintain the natural curve of your lower back and be sure to draw the belly bottom to the spine before and during the exercise.

Paul's Pro Tip

You should be completely comfortable in a two-point perch before attempting this advanced exercise. Practice first with no weights.

TECHNIQUE & FORM

Begin in the two-point perch position. Hold the weights in front of your thighs, keeping your chest high, shoulders back, and maintaining the natural curve of your back. Lower and raise buttocks to heels.

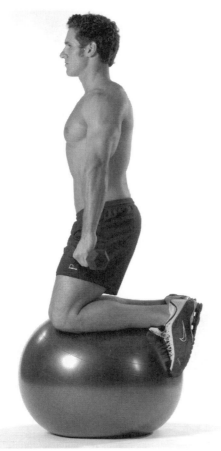
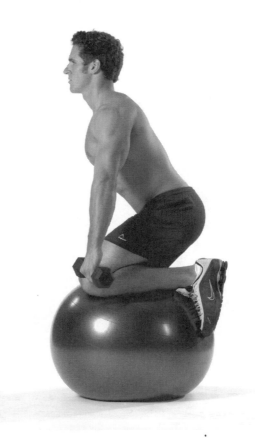

Reverse Back Extension

Concentrate on squeezing the gluteus muscles to lift your legs.

Paul's Pro Tip

Avoid the tendency of swinging your legs to create momentum.

TECHNIQUE & FORM

Place the fitness ball under the front of your hips; place your hands on the floor in front of the ball. Extend your legs behind you, with your feet hip distance apart. Keep a slight bend in your elbows. Slowly lift your legs off of the floor, keeping your knees straight, until your ankles and the back of your head are in a straight line. Your legs should be parallel to your torso, or a bit higher. Hold the position for 3 seconds before returning to the starting position.

VARIATION

Drop your chest toward the floor and bring your legs in line with your torso.

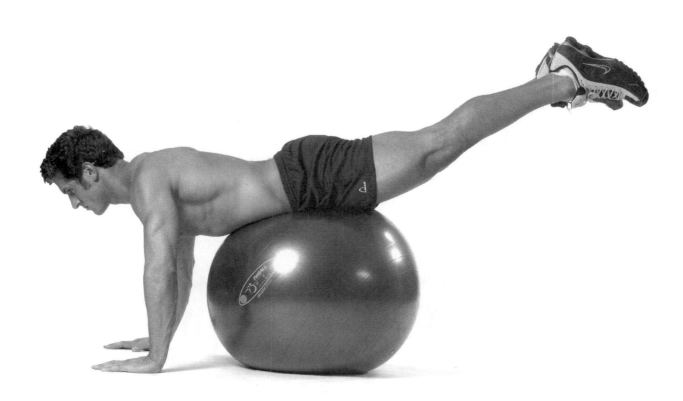

One-Arm Standing Row

The ***One-Arm Standing Row*** is one of the best exercises for the lats (*latissimiss dorsi*). It also doubles as an Arm exercise.

TECHNIQUE & FORM

Place the ball in front of your right foot; place your right hand on the apex of the ball. Bend slightly at the knees. Keep your abdominals tucked in tightly. Hold a weight in your left hand. Let the weight hang with your arm fully extended; keep your shoulder blades back, in a seated position. Pull the weight backward, allowing your elbow to lead the way and sliding your arm along your waist. Repeat on the other side.

VARIATION

This exercise can also train your trunk rotation if you rotate at the waist when lifting the weight.

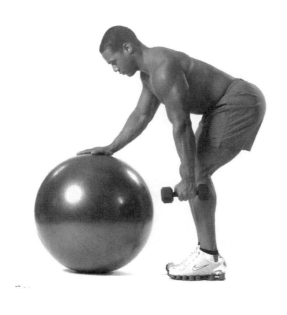

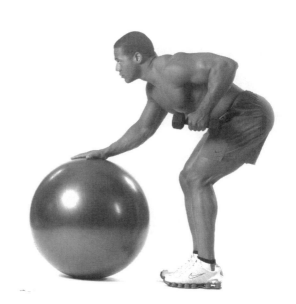

Two-Point Standing Row

The ***Two-Point Standing Row*** is an excellent form of "cross sling training," hitting the upper back and the opposing lower hip and leg.

TECHNIQUE & FORM
Place the ball in front of your right foot; place your right hand on the apex of the ball. Hold a weight in your left hand. Let the weight hang with your arm fully extended; keep your shoulder blades back, in a seated position. Elevate and extend your right leg behind you. Slightly bend your left leg and pull the weight backward, allowing your elbow to lead the way and sliding your arm along your waist. Repeat on the other side.

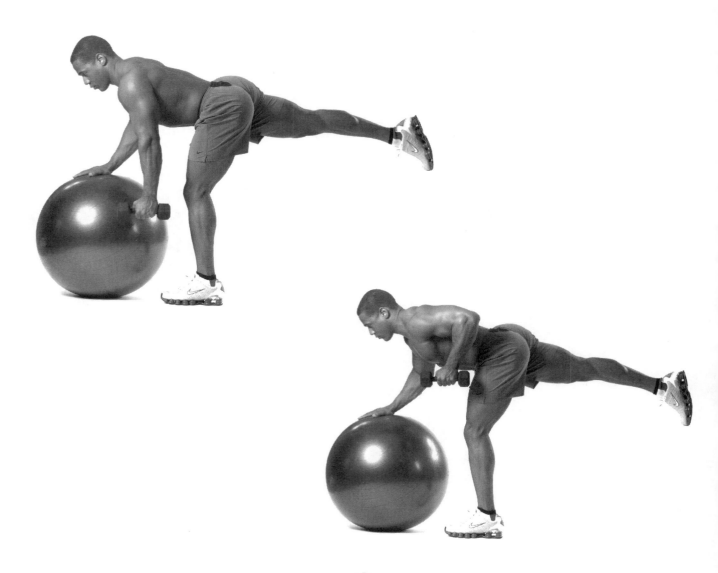

Prone Row

The **Prone Row** targets the upper back and shoulders. Making those muscles strong will correct unattractive forward slouching shoulders and give you a fine straight-back look.

Paul's Pro Tip

When you lie on the ball, make sure you're in a position that doesn't impede your breathing. Avoid the tendency to elevate your shoulders while you do this exercise.

TECHNIQUE & FORM

Lie with your chest on the ball; extend your legs behind you with your feet about shoulder width apart. Hold a dumbbell in each hand. Keeping your chest elevated, pull the weights back with your arms at a 90-degree angle. Keep your shoulders in the seated position and squeeze your shoulder blades together.

VARIATION

Perform the exercise one arm at a time with trunk rotation.

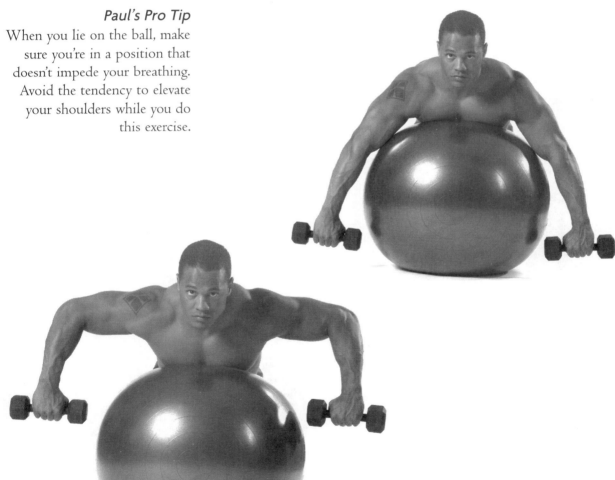

Arm Haulers

Arm Haulers are excellent for strengthening spine extensors and your middle and upper back. Be sure to place the ball where it does not impede your breathing.

TECHNIQUE & FORM

Start with a weight you feel comfortable lifting. Lie with your chest on the ball, your toes on the floor, and the weights at your sides. Keep your head aligned with your spine to avoid stressing your neck. Move the weights from your hips to out in front of you in a circular motion.

VARIATION

These are challenging if you do them with no weight but lots of reps.

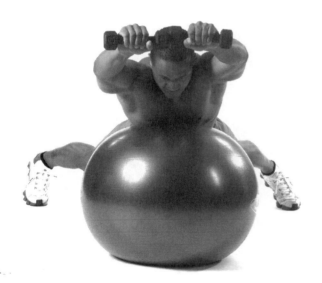

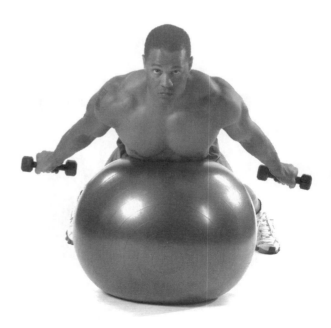

One-Arm Reverse Fly

The **One-Arm Reverse Fly** will target the hard to train rear shoulders. It also trains all the back extensors in reverse extension.

Paul's Pro Tip
Do not allow your hips to drop. Keep them aligned with your spine.

TECHNIQUE & FORM
Lay with your chest on the ball, extending your legs behind you. On your toes with your feet hip distance apart, hold a dumbbell in each hand. Plant one hand firmly on floor and lift the opposing hand diagonally off of the floor. Alternate one side to the other.

VARIATION
Lift the same side-arm and leg at the same time.

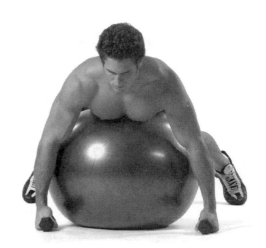

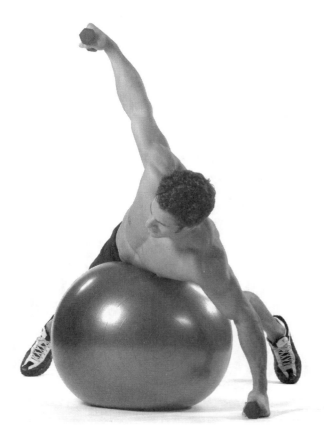

PowerSculpt SHOULDERS

anterior, medial, and posterior deltoids

Strong, sculpted, and square shoulders. Well, to develop powerful and functional shoulders you want to target your shoulder muscles (deltoids) on three different planes: the side (lateral), the rear (posterior), and the front (anterior) of the shoulder. And the exercises on the following pages do just that.

As you perform each of these exercises, keep several points in mind: (1) Always maintain proper shoulder position throughout the full range of motion; (2) Begin with light weights; and (3) Never lift the weight above shoulder height if you have shoulder problems.

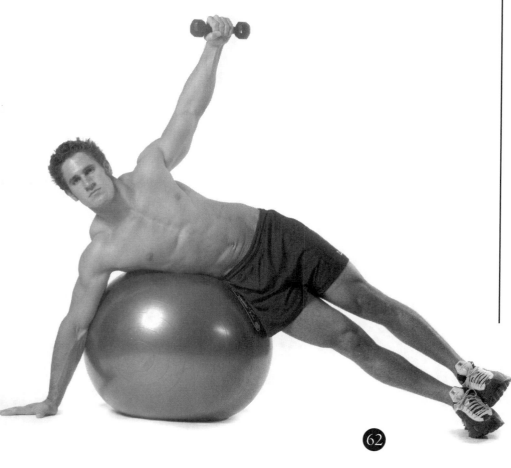

The Exercises

Fly & Hug

The ***Fly & Hug*** takes the usual chest fly to a new level, strengthening the chest and rear shoulders.

Paul's Pro Tip
Do this exercise with a light weight, because your chest muscles will be much stronger than the rear shoulder.

TECHNIQUE & FORM

Sit on the apex of the ball with your feet shoulder width apart. Slowly walk your feet forward, letting the ball roll up your back until it reaches your shoulders. Stop and elevate your hips so that they're parallel to the floor. Your head and neck should be comfortably resting on the ball. Do a chest fly, but instead of stopping when your hands meet in the middle, continue the movement until the weights touch the opposite shoulder.

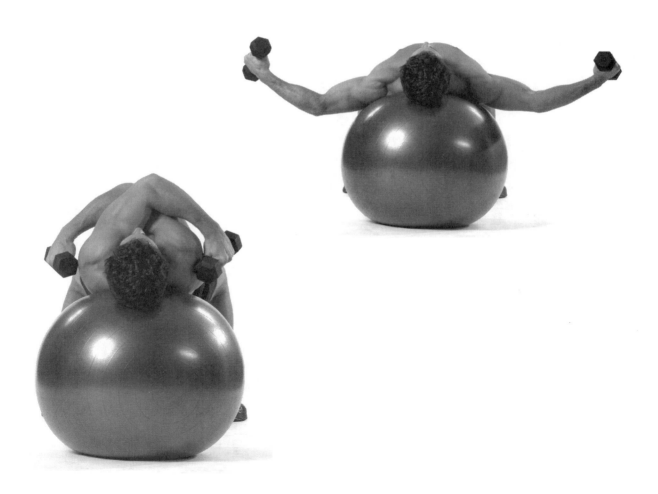

Seated Lateral Raise

TECHNIQUE & FORM

Sit on the apex of the ball. Maintain proper posture and keep your feet flat on the floor. Hold the dumbbells (palms down) by your sides, letting them rest on the side of the ball. Keeping your elbows bent slightly, slowly lift the dumbbells out to your sides and to shoulder height. Lower them, but don't let them rest on the ball again.

Avoid this exercise if you have shoulder problems. Keep your shoulders down and away from your ears.

Paul's Pro Tip
If you prefer, lift or press the weights over your head instead of raising them laterally. Do not allow weights to rest on the ball while in the lowered position.

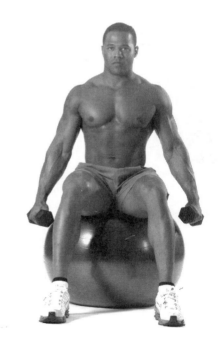

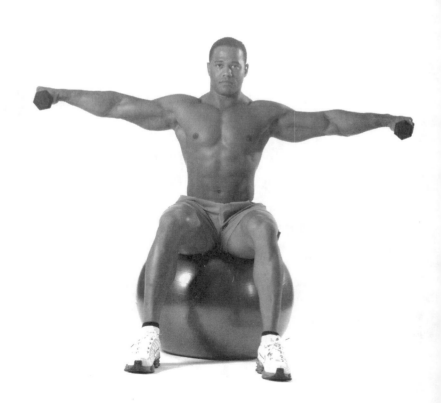

Waist-on-Ball Lateral Raise

You may need to use a smaller ball to do this exercise. You will feel your lower leg working to stabilize your body while in this position.

TECHNIQUE & FORM

Lie with your hips and waist on the ball. The hand of the bottom arm should be flat on the floor. Hold the dumbbell (palms down) by your side. Keeping your elbows bent slightly, slowly lift the dumbbell to shoulder height and then lower it, but don't let it rest on your side again.

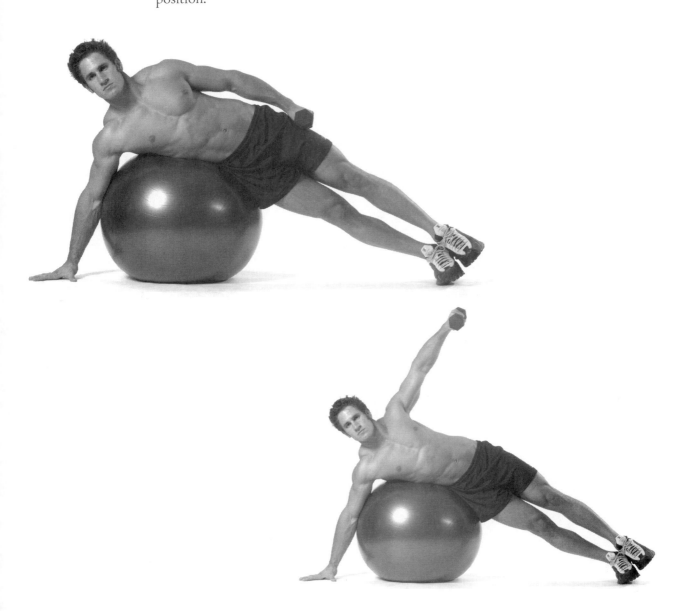

Seated Shoulder Press

The ***Seated Shoulder Press*** works your arms and your shoulders, all while challenging your stability on the ball.

TECHNIQUE & FORM
Sit on the apex of the ball with your chest high and shoulders back. Holding the weights with both hands, press them over your head and then lower them again.

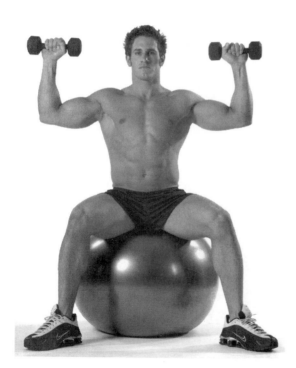

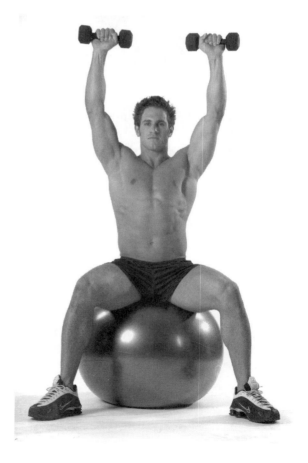

Two-Point Shoulder Press

You should be completely comfortable in a two-point stance on the ball before using weights. Practice with no weights in your hands and then begin with very light weights.

Paul's Pro Tip
This is a very advanced exercise. This should first be done without any weight to establish a movement pattern.

TECHNIQUE & FORM
Hold the weights with your arms bent at 90 degrees. Press the weight over your head, and keep your belly drawn in tight.

VARIATION
Try this exercise with bilateral movements.

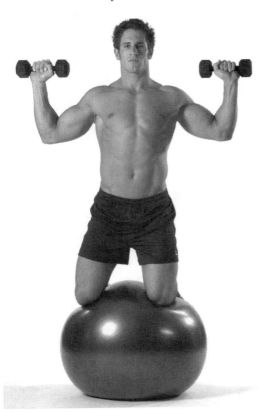

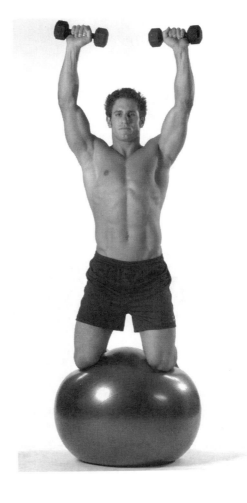

Reverse Fly

TECHNIQUE & FORM

Sit on the apex of the ball. Maintain proper posture and keep your feet flat on the floor. Hold the dumbbells (palms facing inward) by your side. Bend at the waist so that your chest comes close to your knees and the weights are by your ankles. Lift the weights until they're parallel to the floor. Slowly lower them back to the starting position and repeat.

The posterior deltoid is typically the weakest of the three shoulder muscles because it is difficult to isolate. To properly target these rear shoulder muscles, lighten up the weight so you use correct form.

Paul's Pro Tip

Maintain the curve in your lower back. It is essential to keep the belly button drawn in during this exercise.

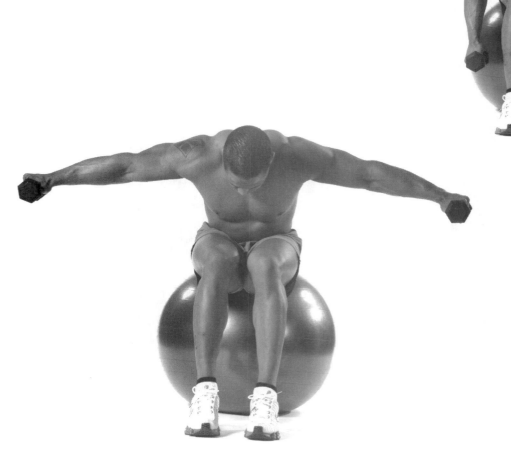

Rear Delts

As with the other waist-on-ball exercises, you may have to switch to a smaller ball to maintain correct form.

Paul's Pro Tip
It is more stable to keep your feet apart.

TECHNIQUE & FORM
Lie with your hips and waist on the ball. The hand of the bottom arm should be flat on the floor. Extend the top arm straight out in front of you, holding the weight palm-down. Keeping your elbows bent slightly, slowly lift the dumbbell over your head and then slowly lower it again.

VARIATION
Lift your top leg to enhance the glutes.

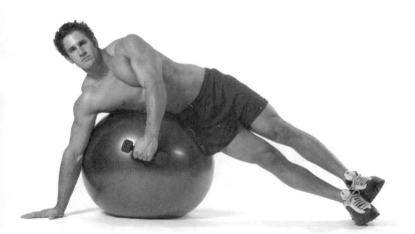

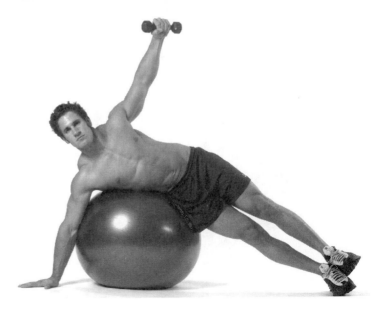

Seated Anterior Raise

To properly execute the *Seated Anterior Raise,* focus on keeping the shoulder blades in a seated position and avoid swinging the weight.

Paul's Pro Tip
Maintaining proper shoulder position throughout the full range of motion is essential. Focus on keeping the shoulders down and in a seated position.

TECHNIQUE & FORM
Sit on the apex of the ball. Maintain proper posture and keep your feet flat on the floor. Hold the dumbbells (palms facing inward) by your side, not letting them rest on the side of the ball. Lift the weights in front of you to shoulder height. Hold for a second before lowering the weights back to the staring position; repeat.

VARIATION
For a more advanced exercise, drop your butt to your heels when lowering the weight. Lift the weight and hips together.

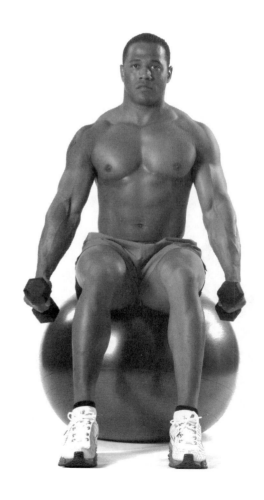
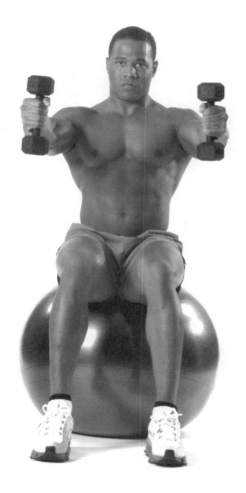

Two-Point Anterior Raise

To perform the *Two-Point Anterior Raise* without losing your balance, it's important to do it slowly.

TECHNIQUE & FORM

Kneel on the apex of the ball. Hold the dumbbells with your palms facing inward. Lift the weights in front of you to shoulder height. Hold for a second before lowering the weights back to the starting position; repeat.

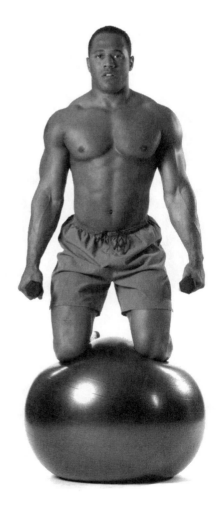

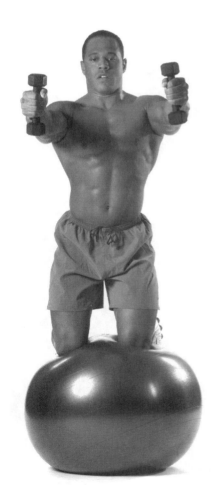

One-Arm Shoulder Snatch

The *One-Arm Shoulder Snatch* is a great way to exercise the shoulders. The lower back, biceps, and shoulders work together. When mastered it can be done standing to engage the legs and butt.

Paul's Pro Tip
Keep the ball stable. Try not to allow it to roll back and forth to accommodate your movement.

TECHNIQUE & FORM
Sit on the apex of the ball. Hold your knees at 90 degrees and your feet flat on the floor. Your chest should be high and your shoulders back, maintaining the curve in your lower back. Hold the weight in one hand, and lower it between both feet by bending at the hips. Then straighten your torso to a sitting position and do a bicep curl. At the top of the bicep curl, press the weight overhead.

VARIATION
Try the One Arm Shoulder Snatch in a Two-Point Perch position. This is a more advanced alternative.

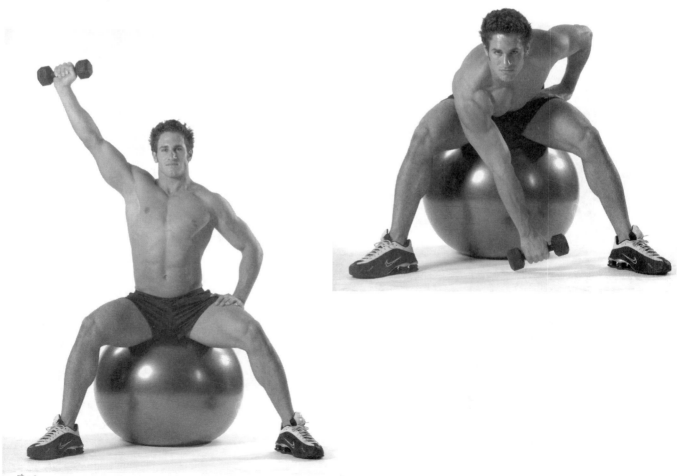

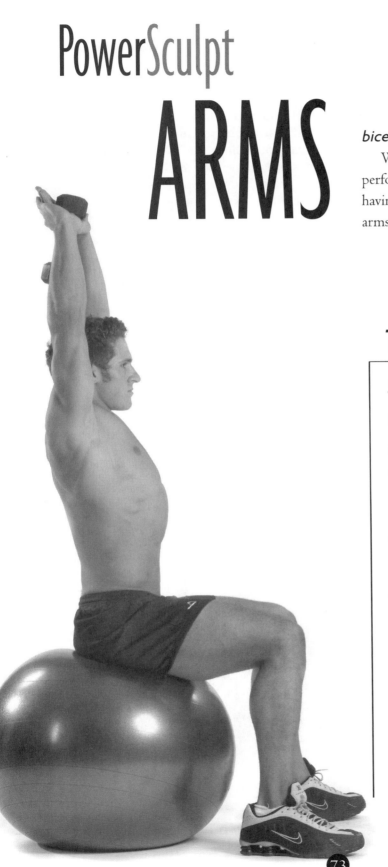

PowerSculpt
ARMS

biceps brachii and triceps brachii

What good are big strong arms if they don't perform as an extension of your trunk? It's like having a gun with no ammo. Get strong, cut arms that perform as well as they look.

The Exercises

Seated Biceps Curl

This is another classic exercise paired with the fitness ball. As your strength and balance improve you'll be able to move to heavier weights—and the *Two-Point Biceps Curls*.

TECHNIQUE & FORM

Start with a weight you feel comfortable lifting. Sit on the apex of the ball with your feet flat on the floor. Keep your chest high and your shoulders back. Let the weights hang by your sides, resting on the ball. Raise the weights with your palms facing your shoulders. Lower them, but don't let them rest on the ball again.

VARIATION

Do the biceps curls with only one foot on the floor. This intensifies the exercise by incorporating your leg and trunk muscles.

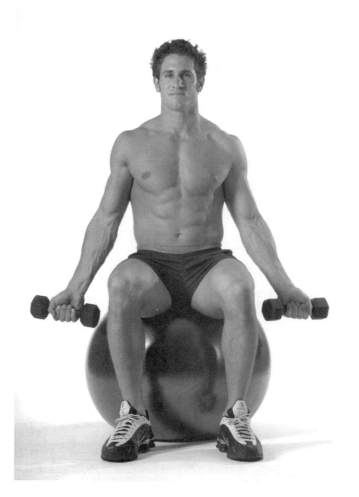
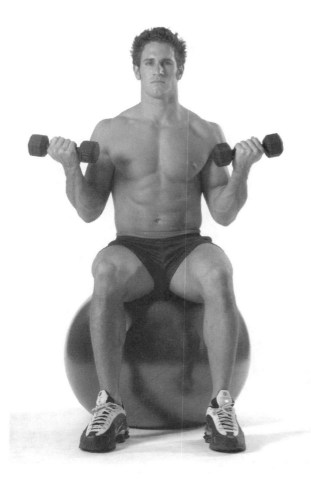

Incline Biceps Curl

Placing the biceps in a stabilized and inclined position on the ball will keep you from cheating with momentum and give the biceps a full stretch before contraction.

TECHNIQUE & FORM

Sit on the apex of the ball and then roll down to the Tabletop position, allowing your lower back to remain on and be supported by the ball. Your elbows and the backs of your upper arms should rest comfortably on the ball. Let the weights hang freely with your arms fully extended; you will most likely feel a stretch of the biceps muscle. Lift the weights toward the top of your shoulders in a full range of motion and then return to the bottom position.

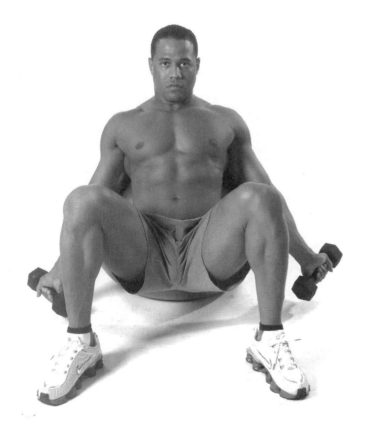
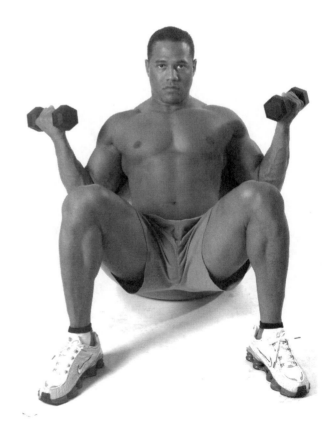

Preacher Curl

The *Preacher Curl* is isolation
with a PowerSculpt twist.

TECHNIQUE & FORM
Start with a weight you feel comfortable lifting. Kneel
behind the ball, resting your triceps on its apex.
Maintain your stability as you perform curls with one or
both arms.

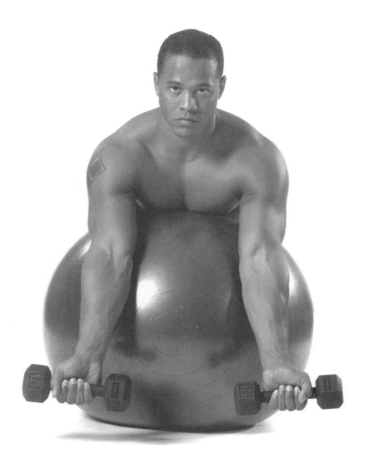
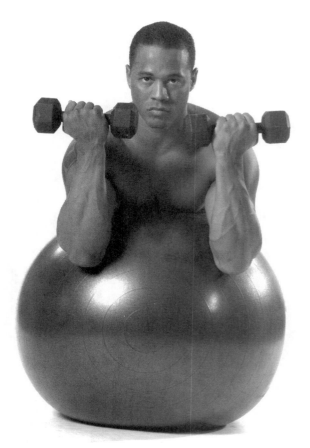

Two-Point Biceps Curl

This is an advanced exercise and one that you shouldn't attempt unless you're completely confident in your ability to maintain a two-point stance on the ball.

TECHNIQUE & FORM

Approach the ball with the weights in your hands. Place your knees and hands on the ball and roll to a four-point stance. Lift yourself to a two-point stance. Maintain stable hips as you do biceps curls. Try curls working one arm at a time and then both arms at once.

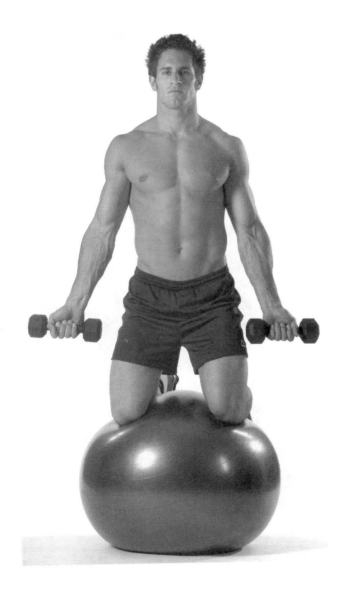

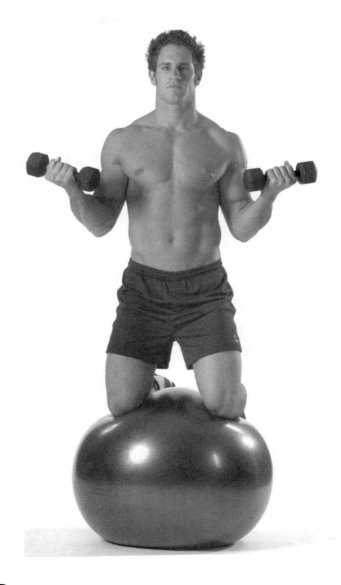

Standing Triceps Extension

This exercise is an old favorite done with the fitness ball. The benefit? In addition to sculpting your triceps, you'll be improving your balance and stability.

TECHNIQUE & FORM

Start with a weight you feel comfortable lifting. Stand with your legs slightly bent, one hand on the ball, and the weight in your free hand. Lift your arm behind you until your upper arm is parallel to the floor. Straighten and bend your elbow.

VARIATION

Lift your opposing leg to be parallel to your trunk to incorporate your hips and legs.

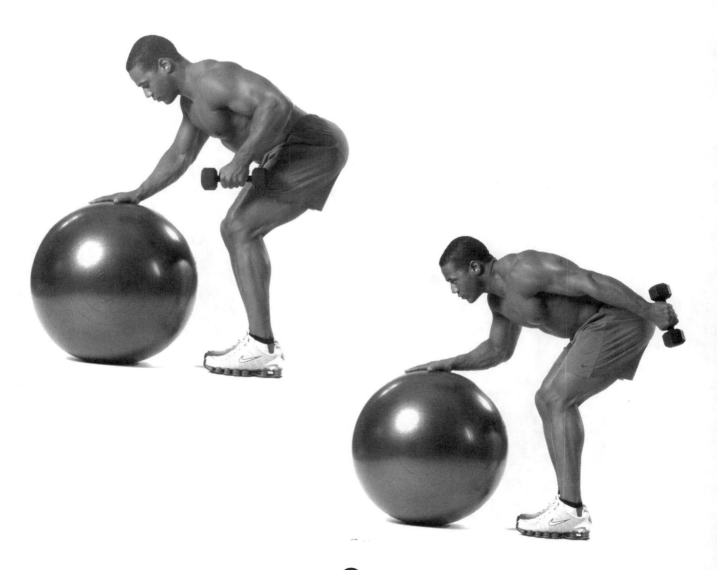

Seated Overhead Triceps Extension

Changing the angle of the triceps extensions targets different muscle fibers.

Paul's Pro Tip

Make sure that you keep your elbows close to your head at all times. Keep your upper arms fixed and elbows pointing up.

TECHNIQUE & FORM

Start with a weight you feel comfortable lifting. Sit on the apex of the ball. Hold the dumbbell with both hands and place it over your head. Keeping the elbows parallel with each other, lower the weight behind your head with your forearms until your elbows are bent at a 90-degree angle. Press up with your forearms using the triceps muscle. Keep the elbows slightly bent in the uppermost position.

VARIATION: Two-Point Triceps Extension

Try this exercise in two-point perch. This is an advanced variation that challenges stability in the sagittal plane.

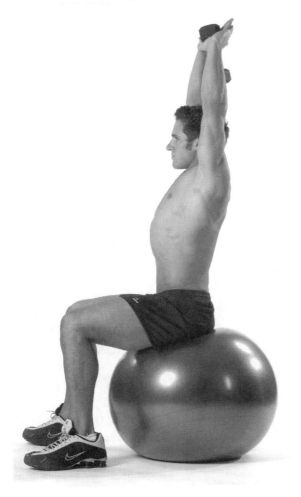
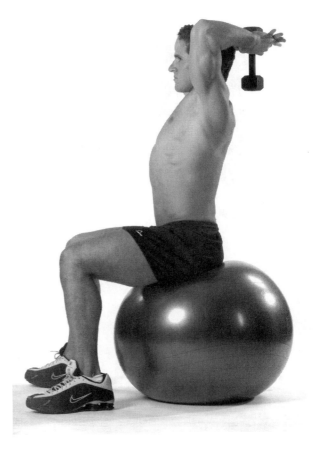

Tabletop Triceps Extension

Anytime you can do an exercise in a tabletop position, you should. Not only are you targeting your triceps, you engage your lower back, butt, hamstring, and core.

TECHNIQUE & FORM

Start with a weight you feel comfortable lifting. Sit on the apex of the ball and roll down to the tabletop position. Once there, extend your arms over your chest. Bend your arm at the elbow, lowering the weights so that they're parallel to the floor.

VARIATION

Change the handgrip so your palms face your head. This will target different muscle groups.

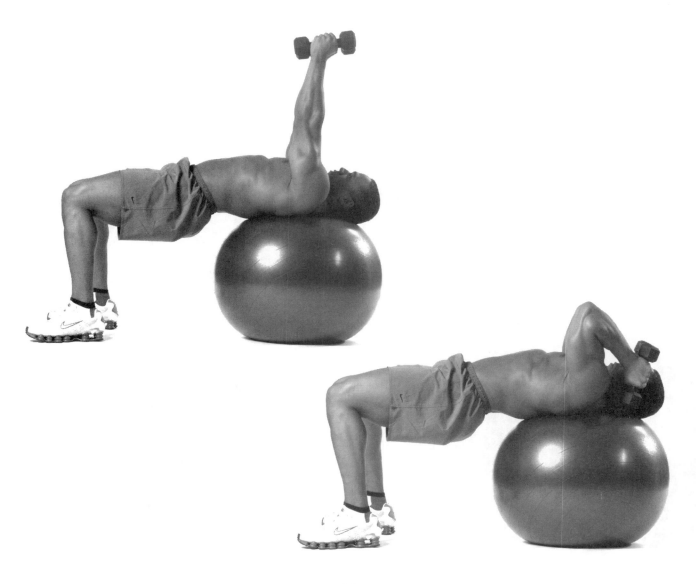

Seated Dip

Another classic triceps exercise updated with the fitness ball!

Paul's Pro Tip

Once you've mastered this one, try it while lifting one leg off the ball.

TECHNIQUE & FORM

Sit on a bench and place your ankles on the ball. Keep your fingers pointed forward, toward the ball. Lift your hips off of the bench and lower your body until your elbows are bent at a 90-degree angle. Raise yourself again.

VARIATION

Sit on the ball and place your hands next to your butt. Lift yourself off the ball and drop your hips toward the floor. Try this with your feet on the floor at first. Placing your feet on the bench is a more advanced option.

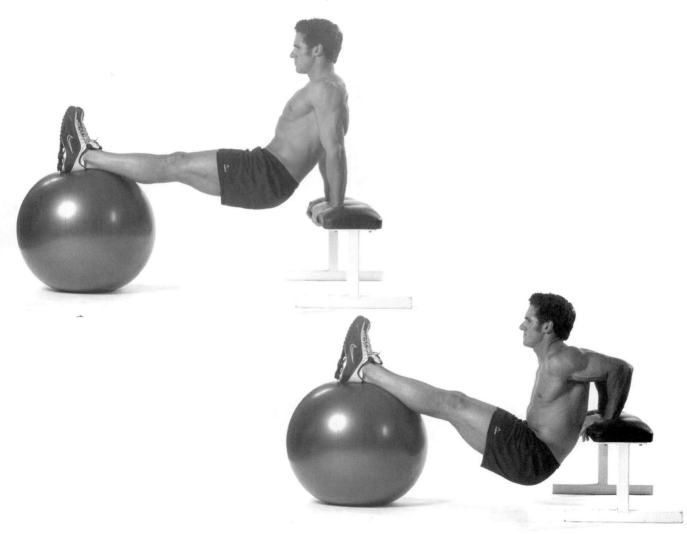

Long Head Press

The **Long Head Press** recruits heavily from your triceps.

Paul's Pro Tip

If you're having trouble balancing, move your feet wider apart. Keep your shoulder blades pressed together tightly to better target your chest muscles.

TECHNIQUE & FORM

Start with a weight you feel comfortable lifting. Sit on the apex of the ball with your feet more than shoulder width apart. Slowly walk your feet forward, letting the ball roll slowly up your back to your shoulders. Stop and elevate your hips so that they're parallel to the floor. Your head and neck should be resting comfortably on the ball and your feet should be flat on the floor. Keeping your shoulder blades back, press the weights up over your chest. Keep the weights in line with your elbows.

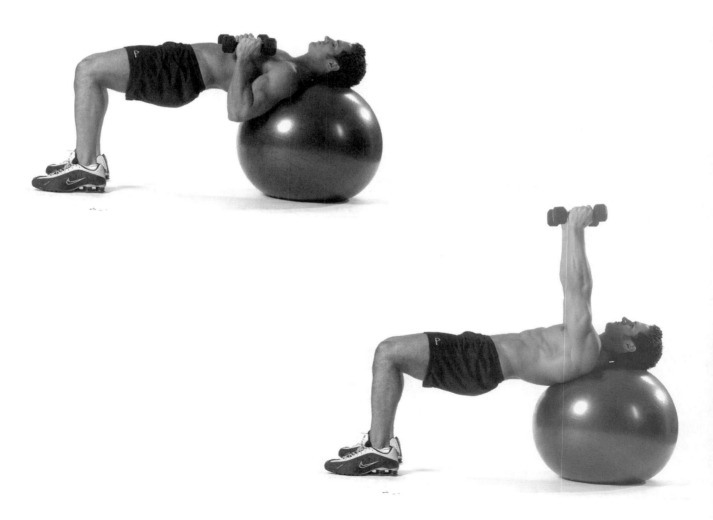

PowerSculpt

ABS

There is no other muscle group like the abs to tell the world how fit and vital you are. We can talk all we want about what exercises we do and the results we get, but talk is cheap. Don't tell me how well your exercise program works and how great it is! Stand up on a table and show me your abs. If you're willing to do that in a room full of your peers, then you have great abs. To properly work your abs, you need to train them using a variety of movements: flexion, extension, and rotation. Training your abs on a fitness ball engages even more muscle fiber in a greater range of motion.

Sure, we want to look good, but we want to be self-confident, too. We want to be self-confident enough to work an eight-hour day and have enough left to pick up our kids, do yard work, sweep our lady off her feet, and have plenty left over for the softball game. If you agree with this, it's important to not ignore your abs.

The Exercises

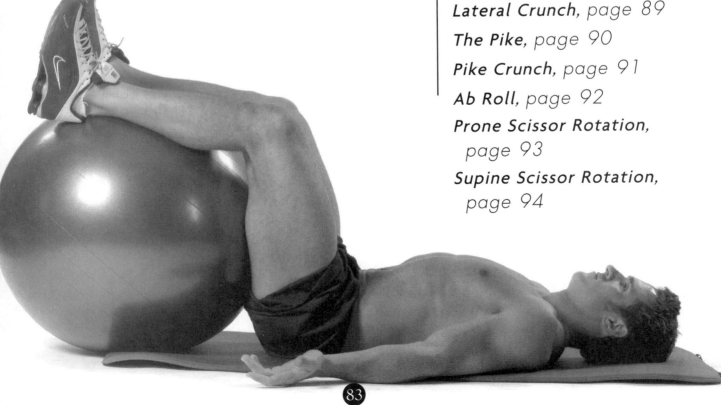

Crunch

Doing crunches on the fitness ball increases the range of motion through which your abs must work. That makes the fitness ball *Crunch* a much more effective exercise.

TECHNIQUE & FORM

Sit on the apex of the ball with your feet shoulder width apart. Walk your feet forward until your lower back is firmly supported. Place your fingers by your temples; keep your elbows wide. Lower your upper back and shoulders onto the ball. Lift your upper back and shoulders off the ball to a roughly 45-degree angle. Keep your hips anchored so that you move over the ball, and the ball does not roll under you. Keep your tongue on the roof of your mouth to assist in engaging your deep neck flexors.

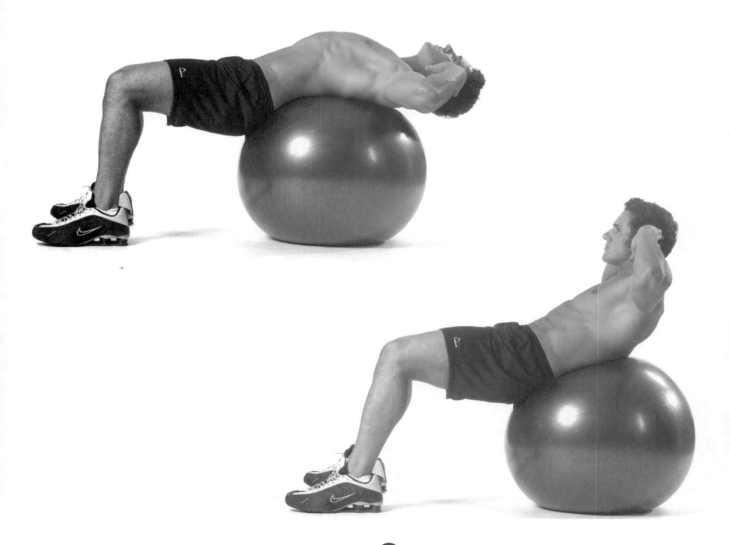

Reverse Crunch

The *Reverse Crunch* targets the hard-to-engage lower abdominals. Placing your legs on the ball while doing the reverse crunch will help disengage the hip flexor and will better target the lower portion of your abs.

Paul's Pro Tip

If you feel discomfort in your lower back, don't lower the ball all the way to the floor.

TECHNIQUE & FORM

Lie on your back on the floor with your knees bent and legs on the ball. The ball should be wedged between your butt and calves. Lift the ball off the floor with your heels and draw your knees to your chest and then slowly return them to the floor.

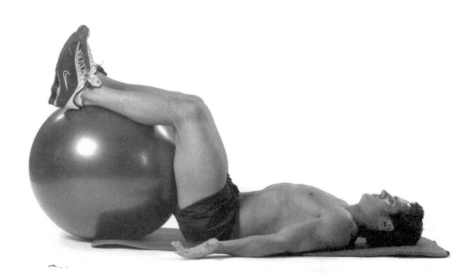

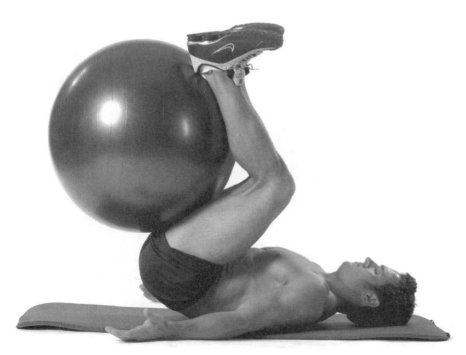

Crunch with Rotation

The *Crunch with Rotation* adds a twist that engages your obliques. Strong obliques are desirable because they strengthen one of the most important and powerful of movements in sports performance: the shoulder-to-hip rotation.

TECHNIQUE & FORM

Sit on the apex of the ball with your feet shoulder width apart. Walk your feet forward until your lower back is firmly supported. Place your fingers by your temples; keep your elbows wide. Lower your upper back and shoulders onto the ball. Lift your upper back and shoulders off the ball to a roughly 45-degree angle. As you do so, turn your torso to the left, and then lower yourself. Repeat, switching sides.

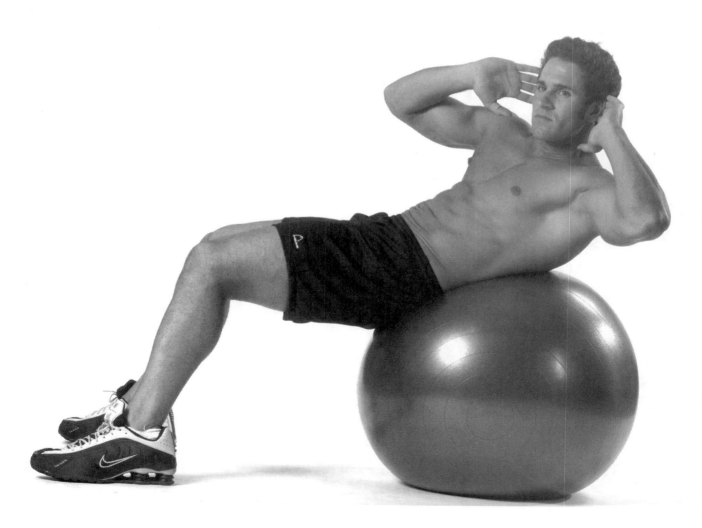

Prone Crunch with Knee Curl

The **Prone Crunch with Knee Curl** strengthens the lower abdominal region and your shoulders. Stabilize your shoulder and initiate the movement by drawing the belly into the spine.

Paul's Pro Tip

It's important to keep your hips elevated while you draw your knees into your chest.

TECHNIQUE & FORM

Lay on your hips on the ball. Walk your hands out until your insteps are on the ball's apex. Pull the ball into your chest and then roll it out again.

VARIATION

Try this one leg at a time.

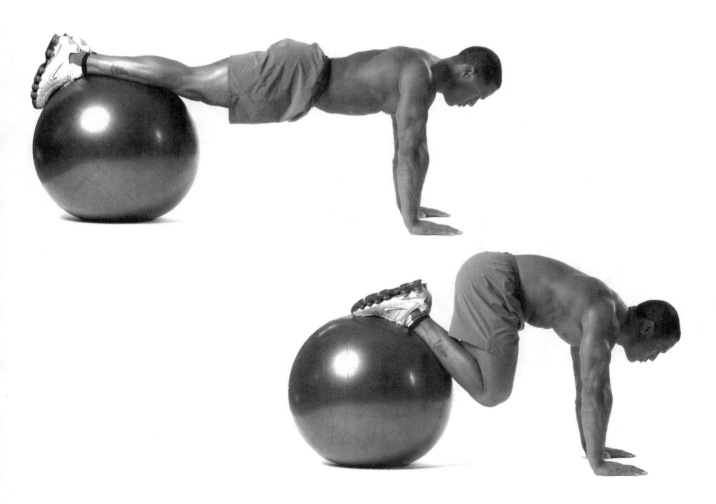

Prone Crunch with Knee Side Curl

This crunch is an excellent exercise for training shoulder stability, core strength, and hip rotation.

TECHNIQUE & FORM
Lay on your hips on the ball. Walk your hands out until your insteps are on the ball's apex. Pull the ball toward one shoulder, then roll it out again. Repeat, moving the ball toward the opposite shoulder.

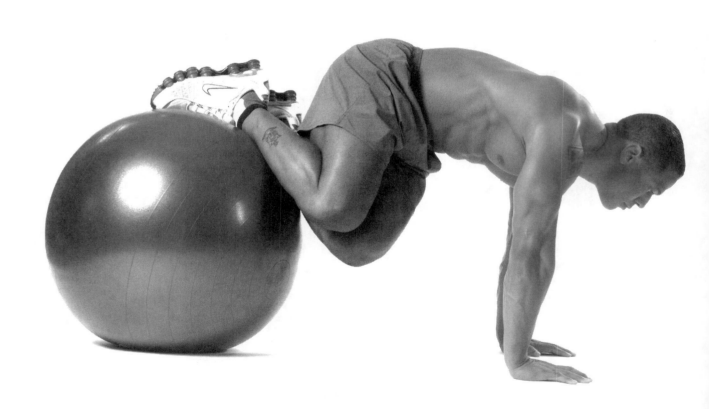

Lateral Crunch

The *Lateral Crunch* is a much-needed, often-ignored abdominal exercise. It targets the internal obliques, which are major stabilizers of the lower back.

Paul's Pro Tip

The size of the ball will increase or decrease the intensity of this exercise. A larger ball gives you a smaller range of motion and is a good place for a beginner to start.

TECHNIQUE & FORM

Place one buttock on the ball with your bottom leg bent at 90 degrees. Your top leg should be straight and its foot can be placed against a wall for stability. Cross your arm across your chest and laterally lower your torso so that your bottom shoulder touches the ball. Hold the torso as if there was a plane of glass in front of you. Avoid rotating.

VARIATIONS

Variation I: Extend your arms to the side or overhead.

Variation II: Hold a weight across your chest.

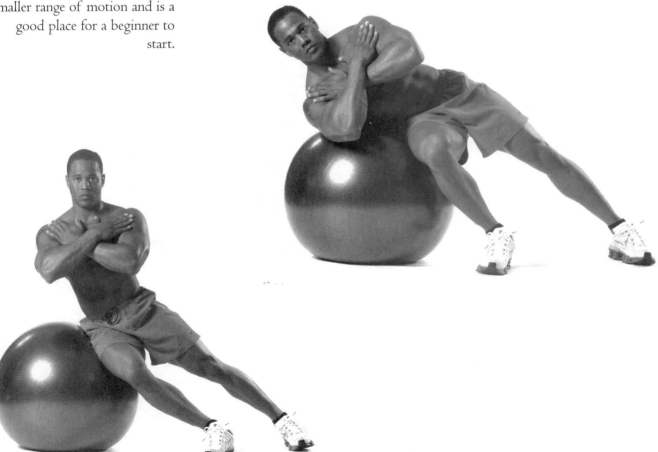

The Pike

Be sure to become very proficient at the crunch with knee curl before attempting *The Pike*! This is a very advanced exercise.

TECHNIQUE & FORM
Lie on the ball and walk your hands out until your ankles are on the ball's apex. Keeping your legs straight, draw the ball toward your hands, but do not bend your knees.

VARIATION
Try this using one leg at a time; this is the single-legged pike.

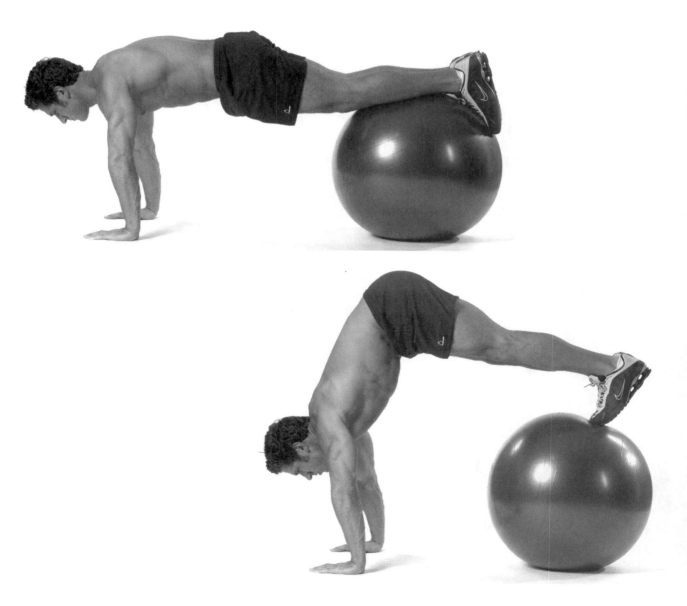

Pike Crunch

TECHNIQUE & FORM

Lie on the floor with the ball between your ankles and your arms extended above your head. Simultaneously lift your shoulder blades and the ball off the floor and transfer the ball from your ankles to your hands. Return to the original position, then repeat.

You will most likely have to work up to this exercise. If you cannot keep your lower back firmly on the floor, then place the ball between your knees, already bent at 90 degrees.

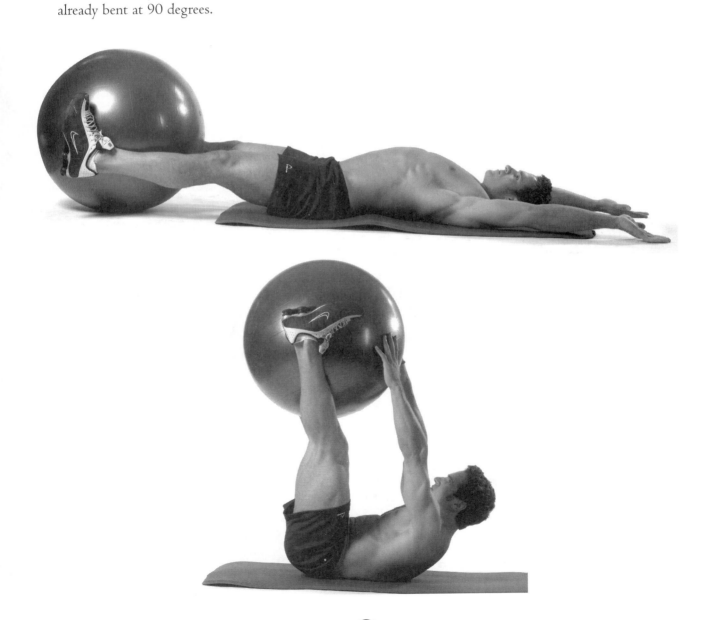

Ab Roll

The **Ab Roll** is an advanced move that will challenge both your abs and your lower back. This exercise may not be appropriate for anyone with shoulder or lower back issues.

Paul's Pro Tip
It's a good idea with this, or any exercise in the prone position, to start with a posterior tilt to protect your back.

TECHNIQUE & FORM
Kneel in front of the ball. Place your forearms on the ball's apex with your fingers interlaced. Roll the ball forward until your arms, hips, and knees are in a straight line. Do not allow your belly to drop.

VARIATION
Try this on your toes in a push-up position.

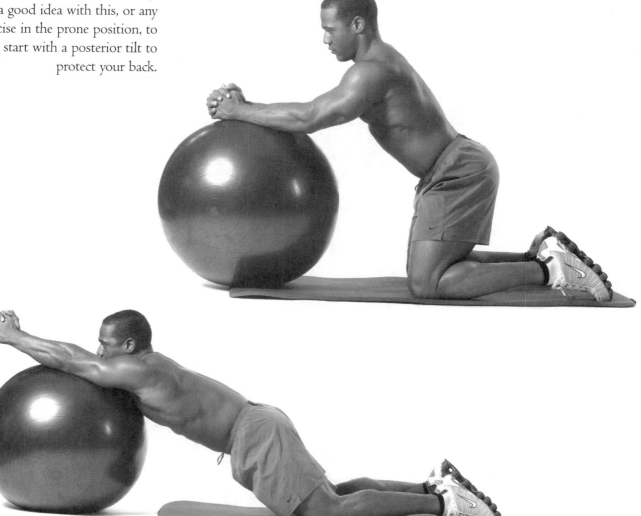

Prone Scissor Rotation

The ***Prone Scissor Rotation*** focuses on your core musculature, but is a full body exercise. It engages the chest, shoulders, legs, and back and is much more functional than many pieces of equipment used in a gym.

Paul's Pro Tip

This is an advanced exercise, but its intensity can be decreased by simply getting into the start position, drawing the belly to the spine, and moving the ball in increments of inches.

TECHNIQUE & FORM

Place your ankles slightly to the side of the top of the ball. Your hands should be shoulder width apart on the floor. Make sure you keep your body aligned. Brace your abdominals and then slowly rotate the ball from side to side. Begin with a small arc and increase your range of motion. Do not allow your hips to sag.

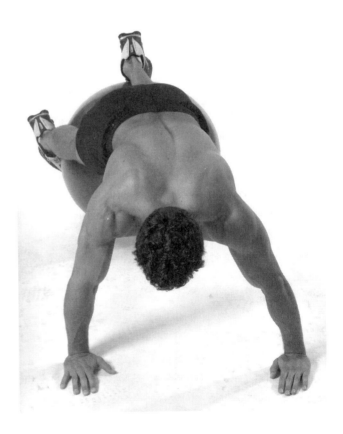

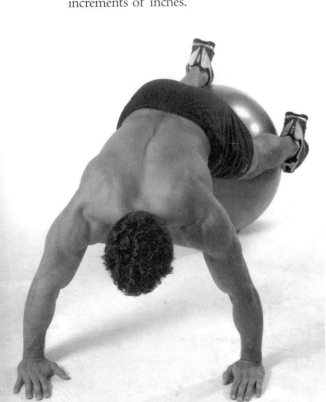

Supine Scissor Rotation

The *Supine Scissor Rotation* is not only core specific, but will also target the extensor chain of your lower back, buttocks, and hamstrings.

TECHNIQUE & FORM

Lay on your back with your ankles on top of the ball. Your arms should be by your side, palms facing up. Elevate your hips so that your shoulders, hips, and ankles are aligned. Begin the exercise by bracing the abdominals. Rotate the ball in a small arc, slowly increasing the range of motion.

Paul's Pro Tip

The extensor chain of lower back, buttocks, and hamstrings works in synergy. The exercise should be felt in all three areas, plus the abdominals. If you feel the exercise only in one area it could be because the other muscles are not yet engaged.

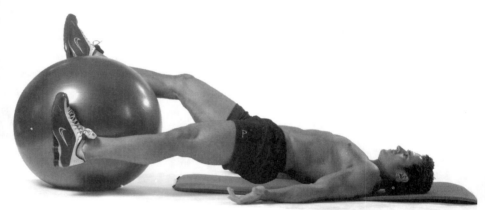

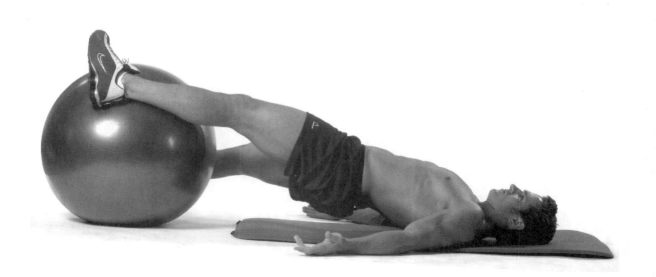

PowerSculpt

LEGS

abductors, adductors, hamstrings, quadriceps, calves

Have you heard this saying about an athlete? "He was good until his wheels went bad." His wheels being his legs. Developing strong legs is the stability, base, and foundation, from which all athletic movements derive. From boxing to golfing to horseshoes, if it's a sport which requires being on your feet, it requires you to have strong legs.

The Exercises

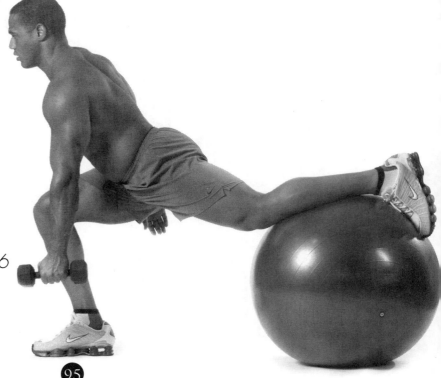

Wall Squat

Using the fitness ball in this fashion teaches a beginner proper form for squats. (*quadriceps, rectus femoris, vastus lateralis, vastus medialis, vastus intermedius*).

Paul's Pro Tip
Your foot position may vary according to the flexibility level of your ankle, knee, back, or hip. However, be careful not to compromise your posture to achieve a greater range of motion. Accommodate your range of motion accordingly.

TECHNIQUE & FORM
Stand in front of a wall with your feet at least shoulder width apart. Place the ball between your lower back and the wall. You should be far enough from the wall so that when you squat, your knees don't go beyond your toes. Keep your heels firmly on the ground. Slowly lower your butt to the level of your knees (the back of your thighs should be parallel to floor) and then slowly return to the starting position.

VARIATION
Hold a set of weights at your shoulders as you lower and raise yourself.

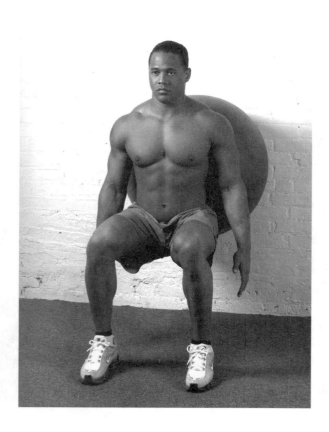

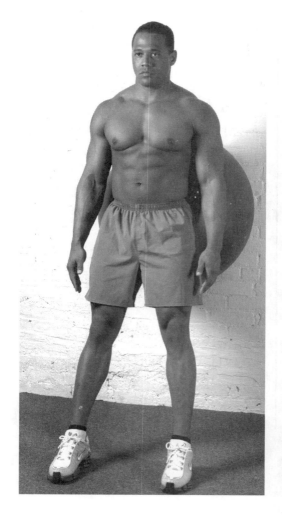

Single-Leg Squat

TECHNIQUE & FORM

Stand in front of a wall with your feet at least shoulder width apart. Place the ball between your lower back and the wall. Lift one foot off the floor and lower yourself until the planted thigh is almost parallel to the floor. Slowly raise yourself again.

VARIATIONS

Variation I: Vary the position of the free leg. It will recruit more lower abs and hip flexor of the free leg. You can also try pointing the free leg in several different directions to further challenge your balance

Variation II: Hold dumbbells in each hand to increase the load.

Begin with 1/4 squats and slowly increase your range of motion.

Paul's Pro Tip

Be sure to line up your standing leg with the center of your body, not directly under the matching hip.

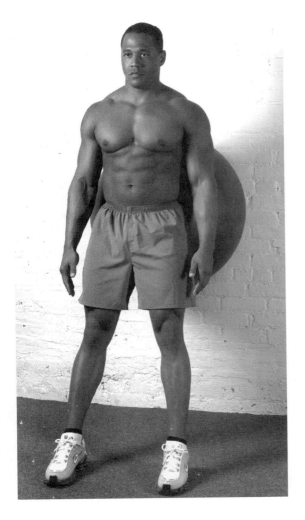

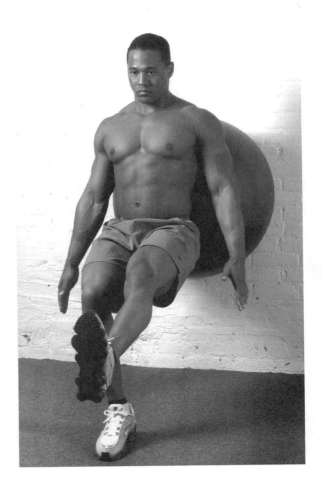

Front Wall Slide

The *Front Wall Slide* is an excellent exercise to combine with the *Seated Calf Raise*. Although they work all the leg muscles, this exercise will give a greater focus on the lower leg muscles.

Paul's Pro Tip
As you become stronger, increase the lean against the ball.

TECHNIQUE & FORM
Place the ball against the wall at your waist height. Press up against the ball, leaning about 60 to 70 degrees. As you squat down, bring your hips back. Your heels should be lifted off of the floor.

VARIATION
Try the single-leg wall slide and start with a higher ball position.

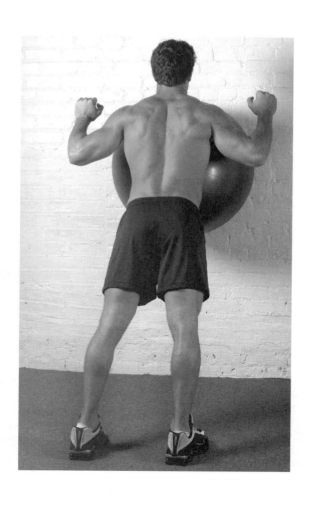

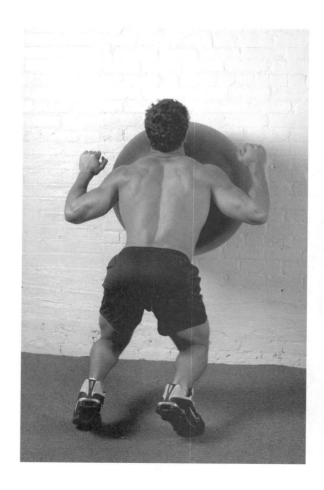

Lateral Wall Slide

The *Lateral Wall Slide* is excellent for developing lateral stability, and creating the strength needed for sports which require changes in direction.

Paul's Pro Tip
Squatting no more than 90 to 100 degrees is optimal.

TECHNIQUE & FORM

Place the ball against the wall with it supporting your body weight at the armpit area. Extend your arms, making contact with the ball in front of you. The initial lean against the ball should be around 70 degrees; the steeper the lean, the more difficult the exercise. Keep your knees and feet together and lower your hips at a 90-degree angle.

VARIATIONS

Variation I: Extend your inside leg behind your hip and balance only on the outside foot.

Variation II: Flex the hip of your outside leg and balance only on the inside foot.

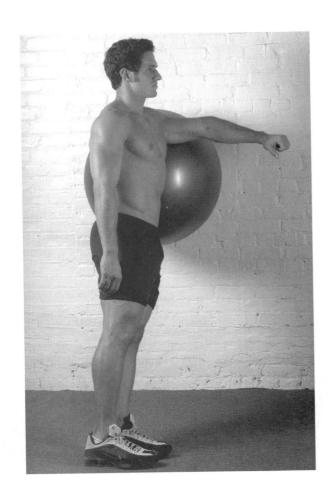

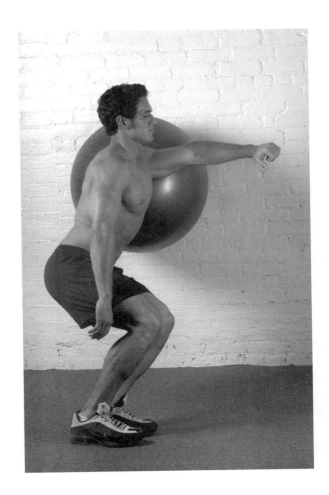

Lunge & Roll

The *Lunge & Roll* is one of the best overall exercises for the legs and glutes.

Paul's Pro Tip

When you do this exercise, you can hold your hands down by your sides or out to the side to aid your balance. You can even brace yourself against a wall with one hand if you need to.

TECHNIQUE & FORM

Stand with your feet shoulder width apart. Place your right instep on the ball behind you. Your knees should be parallel and the standing leg should be bent slightly. You can hold your hands out to the sides for more balance. Bend the standing leg and, at the same time, roll the ball backward with your foot. Lower yourself until the thigh of the lunging leg is almost parallel to the floor. As you straighten the front leg, roll the ball back to the original position.

VARIATION

Increasing the size of the ball will increase your free leg's hip flexors and flexibility.

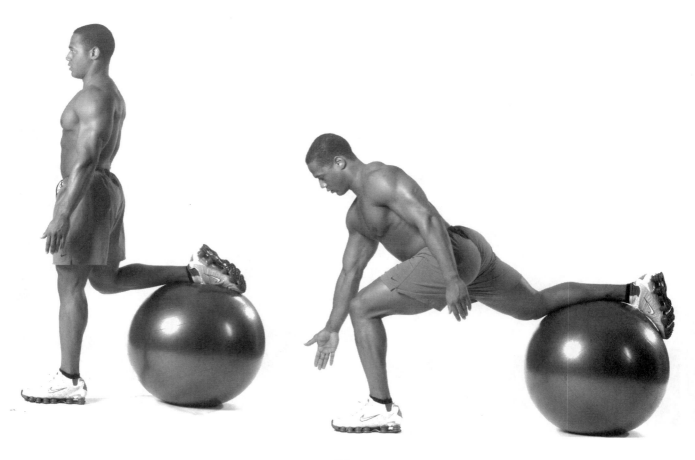

Advanced Lunge & Roll

You may have to work up to this advanced exercise.

Paul's Pro Tip

As you lower and raise yourself, it's important to maintain the natural curve of your lower back.

TECHNIQUE & FORM

Start with a weight you feel comfortable lifting. Stand with your feet shoulder width apart. Place your left instep on the ball behind you. Hold the weight in your left hand. Bend the standing leg and, at the same time, roll the ball backward with your foot. At the same time, lower the weight toward the floor. Lower yourself until the thigh of the lunging leg is almost parallel to the floor. As you straighten the front leg, roll the ball back to the original position.

VARIATION

Do a single-arm row before returning to the standing position.

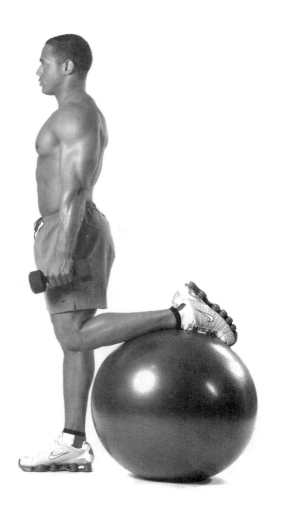

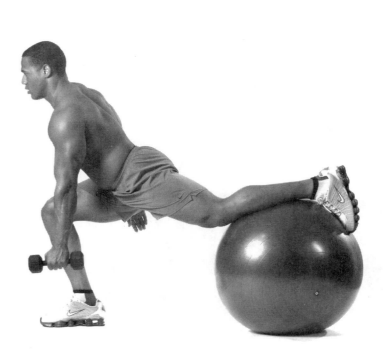

The Lift

TECHNIQUE & FORM

Lay on the ball on your hip, keeping your legs stacked one on top of the other. Be sure to keep the bottom leg firm and place the hand of your bottom arm on the floor for stability. Keep your trunk firm, and do not allow the hips to tip forward or backward. Keep the body in a frontal plane. Lift your top leg and hold.

VARIATIONS

Variation I: Inner Thigh Flex

Bend your top leg to 45 degrees and place your foot on floor. Lift your bottom leg off of the floor.

Variation II: Flex and Kick

With your top leg lifted, bring your knee toward your chest and then press your foot away. Keep your top leg lifted and kick at a 45 degree angle.

The inner and outer thighs might not be a high priority, but they should be. Conditioning of adductors (inner thigh muscles) and abductors (outer thigh group) are important for hip stability and preventing injuries.

Paul's Pro Tip

When practicing **The Lift**, tip your heel toward the ceiling. You will target the glutes. Pointing the toes up will target the quads. Try doing all three exercises one after the other. You will be surprised at how hard the stabilizing leg needs to work.

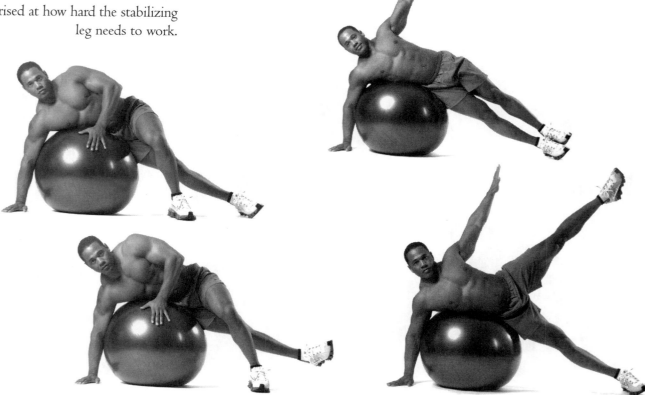

Hamstring Curl

The *Hamstring Curl* targets the muscles of your hamstrings: the *biceps femoris, semitendinosus,* and the *semimembranosus,* which most people neglect.

Paul's Pro Tip
Avoid snapping your knee joint when you do this exercise; keep your knees soft.

TECHNIQUE & FORM
Lay face-up on the floor; place your ankles on top of the ball with your legs together. Keep your hips, shoulders, and head relaxed and on the floor. Extend your arms to your sides. Elevate your hips so that your ankles and shoulders are parallel, forming a straight diagonal line. Keeping your hips elevated, roll the ball in toward your butt. Roll the ball back out and then lower your hips to the floor. Move in a smooth, controlled manner: Elevate the hips, curl in, curl out, lower the hips.

VARIATION
Changing arm positions will challenge your stability: Placing your arms at your sides is a bit more difficult. Cross them across your chest for an even more advanced variation.

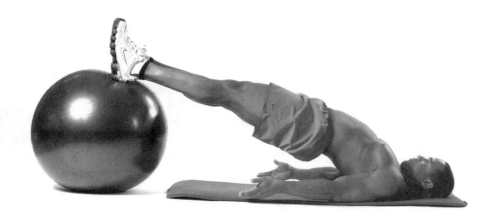

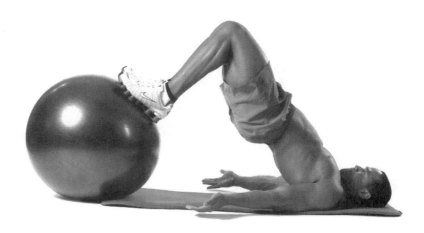

Single-Leg Lateral Ball Squat

The *Single-Leg Lateral Ball Squat* is an excellent exercise to master for anyone that participates in sports which require multi-directional movements.

TECHNIQUE & FORM

Place one foot on top of the fitness ball. Gently roll the ball laterally away as your standing leg moves down into a squat. Keep your torso as upright as possible to engage your core musculature.

VARIATION

Move into the squat position. With the freestanding leg, try to write the alphabet with the ball.

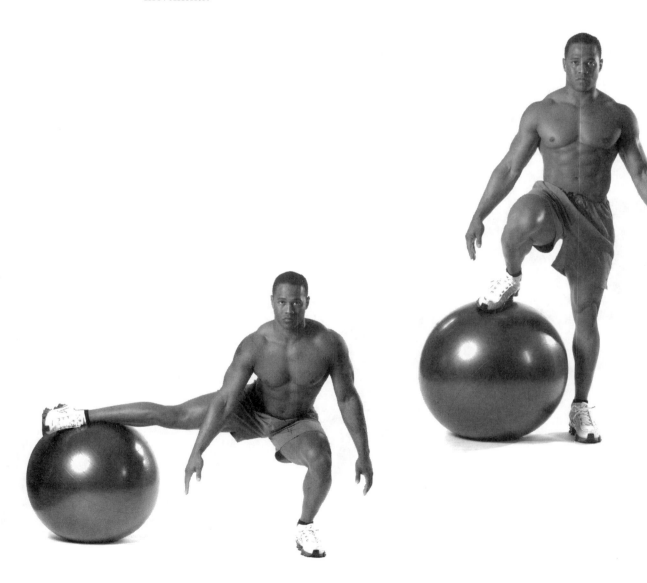

Single-Leg Curl

The *Single-Leg Curl* strengthens the backs of the legs, the glutes, and back. They also develop trunk and hip stability and balance.

TECHNIQUE & FORM

Lay face-up on the floor with your ankles on top of the ball and your legs together. Keep your hips, shoulders, and head relaxed and on the floor. Extend your arms (with palms down) at a 90-degree angle to your sides. Lift one leg straight up off the ball. With the other leg, roll the ball in toward your butt and then roll it back out and place the lifted leg back on the ball. Don't drop your hips back to the floor until you've completed the set; switch legs.

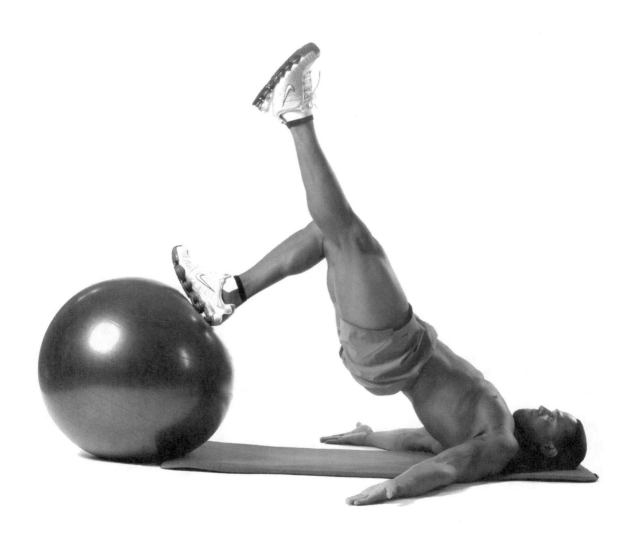

Seated Calf Raise

The **Seated Calf Raise** targets the soleus muscle on the outside section of the lower leg. No lower-leg exercise is complete without training the soleus.

Paul's Pro Tip
Be sure not to place the weight on top of the knee cap.

TECHNIQUE & FORM

Sit on the apex of ball with your feet shoulder width apart and flat on the floor. Place the weights on top of the lower portion of your thighs. Lift your heels off of the floor.

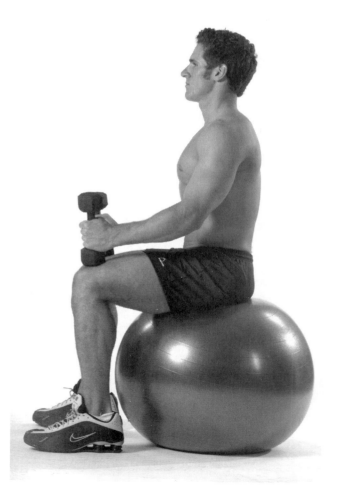
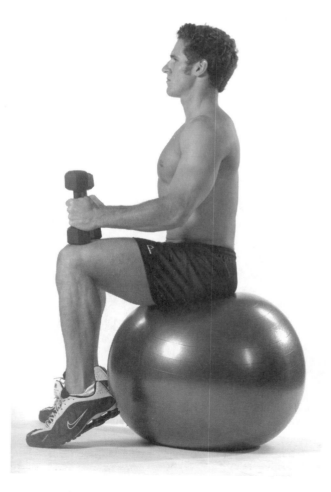

PowerSculpt
GLUTES

gluteus maximus, medius, minimus

What do all great athletes have in common? A "big house." The "big house" means the glutes—the butt or booty. These big boys are responsible for jumping, stopping, switching directions, shifting weight, and explosive forward movements. That's a reason why tough guys are known as "hard asses." A more shallow reason to have strong glutes is they are very attractive to the opposite sex.

The Exercises

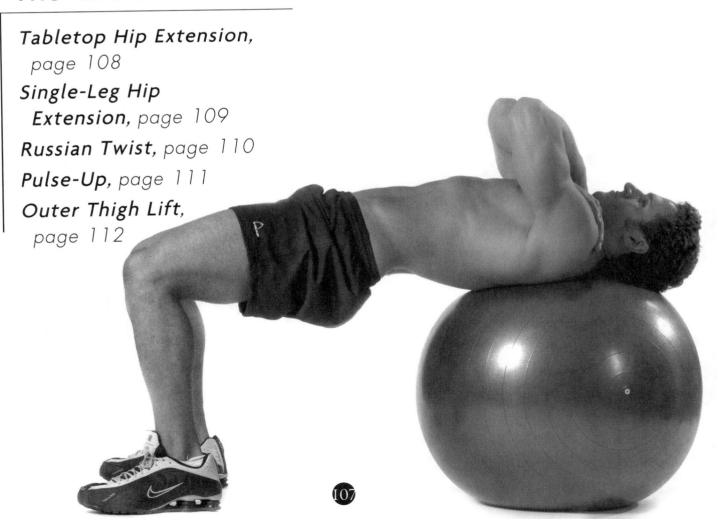

Tabletop Hip Extension

The **Tabletop Hip Extension** trains the butt, the back of the legs, and lower back. It also develops trunk stability.

Paul's Pro Tip
Take care not to hyperextend in the topmost position, and modify the range of motion if you feel any lower back pain.

TECHNIQUE & FORM
Sit on the apex of the ball with your feet shoulder width apart. Slowly walk your feet forward, letting the ball roll up your back until it reaches your shoulders. Your head and neck should be comfortably resting on the ball and your butt should be close to the floor. Press your hips up so that they are parallel to your knees and then lower your hips to the ball again.

VARIATION
Place a barbell plate on your hips to increase the intensity.

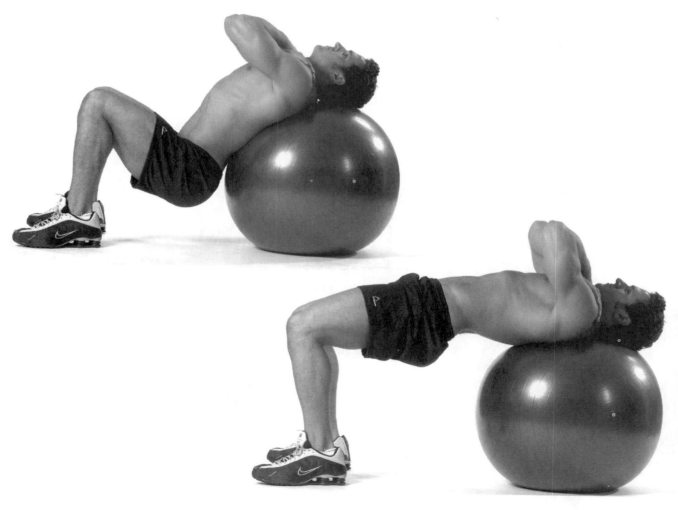

Single-Leg Hip Extension

The ***Single-Leg Hip Extension*** is an advanced and challenging exercise. It develops cross-body stability and balance.

TECHNIQUE & FORM

Sit on the apex of the ball with your feet shoulder width apart. Slowly walk your feet forward, letting the ball roll up your back until it reaches your shoulders. Your head and neck should be comfortably resting on the ball and your butt should be close to the floor. Lift one leg and extend it so that it's parallel to the floor. Stabilize yourself with the grounded foot. Keeping your hips square, press them up so that they are parallel to your knees. Slowly lower your hips back to the ball.

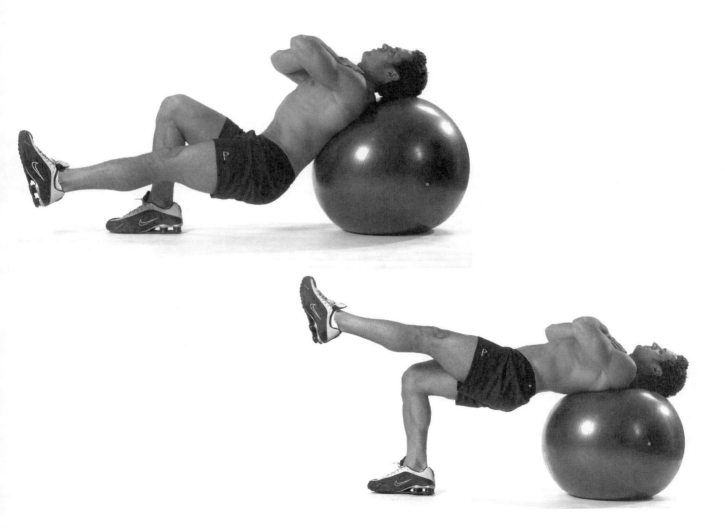

Russian Twist

A good deal of body control is required to do the *Russian Twist.* It not only trains the glutes but also the waist, back, abs, and legs.

Paul's Pro Tip

You will need to constantly adjust your foot position because the fitness ball will slowly move backward.

TECHNIQUE & FORM

Start with a weight that you feel comfortable lifting. Sit on the apex of the ball with your feet shoulder width apart. Slowly walk your feet forward, letting the ball roll up your back until it reaches your shoulders. Stop and elevate your hips so that they're parallel to the floor. Your head and neck should be comfortably resting on the ball. Hold the weight with both hands directly over your chest with both arms extended. With both legs firmly planted on the floor, rotate your torso to the left until the weight is parallel to the floor. Quickly change directions and rotate to the right. Continue rotating from left to right, keeping your abdominals tight and your hips elevated.

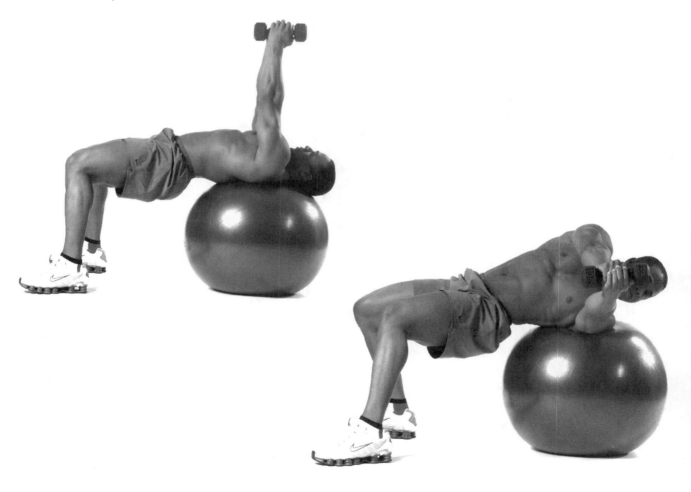

Pulse-Up

The **Pulse-Up** forces you to concentrate on squeezing your glutes.

Paul's Pro Tip
Avoid rocking on the ball as you perform the exercise.

TECHNIQUE & FORM

Lay your hips on the ball's apex. Your hands should be on the floor and your legs hip distance apart with your toes touching the floor. Lift your legs until they're parallel to the floor, and then bend your knees so that the soles of your feet are facing the ceiling. Keeping that position, pulse your legs upward. Imagine that you're pressing the soles of your feet into the ceiling. Focus on tightening the gluteus as you pulse. Don't arch your back. Pulse for the required number of reps, then slowly lower your legs to the starting position.

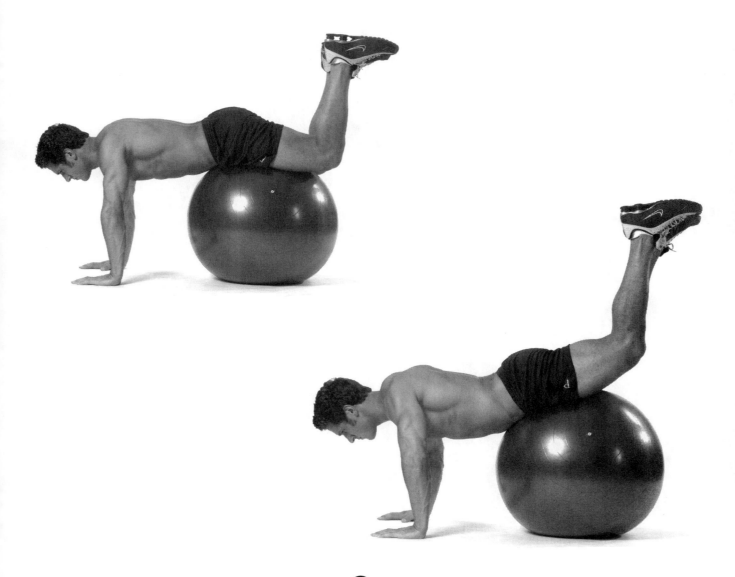

Outer Thigh Lift

By changing the angles at which you lift your legs, you will target different parts of your hips and glutes.

Paul's Pro Tip
Keep the foot on the working leg flexed and the toe pointing toward the floor to keep this exercise focused on the butt.

TECHNIQUE & FORM
Lie on the ball on your hip with your legs stacked. Extend the top leg in front of you at a 45-degree angle. Lower and lift the leg, keeping your foot flexed.

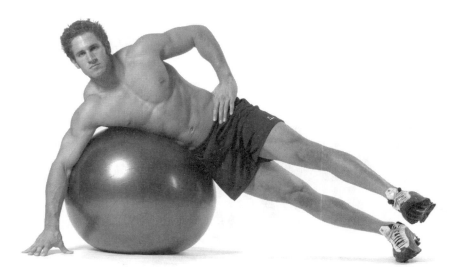

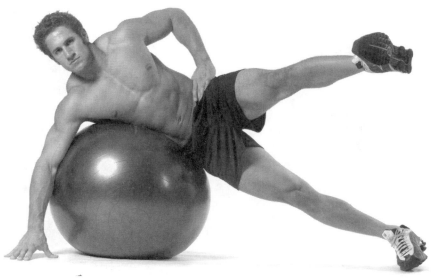

PowerSculpt NECK

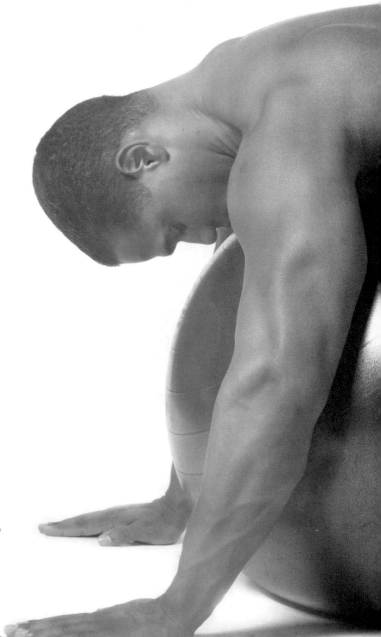

scalenus (anterior, medius, posterior) and sternocleidomastoid

Most of us ignore our neck muscles—that is, until we go out for a long bike ride or feel our necks burn while doing crunches in an aerobics class. These simple exercises will not only give you a lovely neck, but they'll strengthen your neck and reduce stress and neck tension.

The Exercises

Neck Extension

TECHNIQUE & FORM

Lay face down on the ball with your chest on the ball and your feet shoulder width apart. Raise your chin off the ball until your neck is in alignment with your spine and then return to the starting position.

VARIATION

With the ball against the wall, place the back of your head against it. Keep both your head and body aligned. Gently press your head against the ball and hold for 30 seconds.

Paul's Pro Tip

Be sure to give your neck a gentle downward stretch after the neck extension.

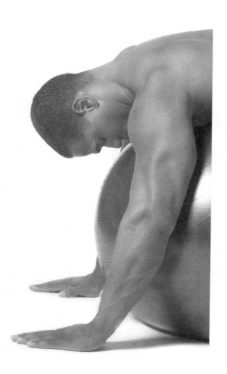

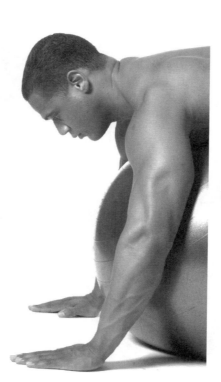

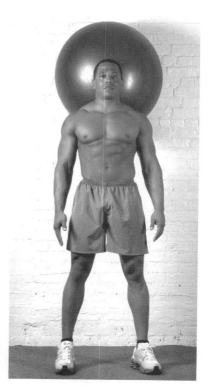

Neck Flexion

This is the exercise that will strengthen your neck so that it doesn't hurt when you do crunches.

Paul's Pro Tip
Do *not* do this exercise if it makes you dizzy.

TECHNIQUE & FORM
Sit on the apex of the ball, with your feet shoulder width apart. Slowly walk your feet forward, letting the ball roll up your back until it reaches your shoulders. Raise your head off the ball and then lower it to the original position.

VARIATION
With the ball against the wall, place your forehead against it. Keep your head and body aligned. Gently press front of head against the ball and hold for 10 to 30 seconds.

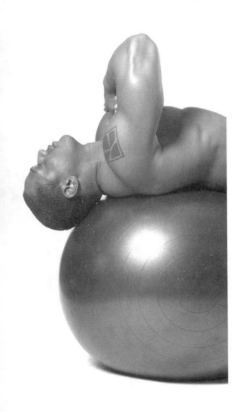

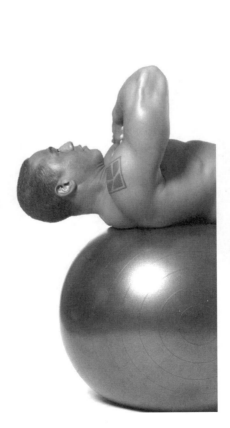

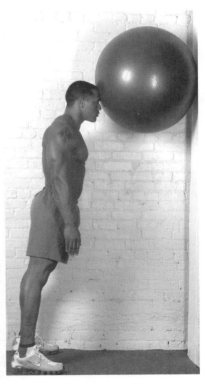

Lateral Neck Press

This one works the side of your neck—you may have never worked those!

TECHNIQUE & FORM

Place the ball against a wall. Get down on your hands and knees and place the side of your head against the ball. Press the ball against the wall with the side of your head. Hold for 3 seconds and then release. Repeat several times. Do both your left and right sides.

VARIATION

With the ball against the wall, place the side of your head against the ball. Keep your head and body aligned. Gently press the side of your head against the ball and old for 10 to 30 seconds. Repeat for the other side.

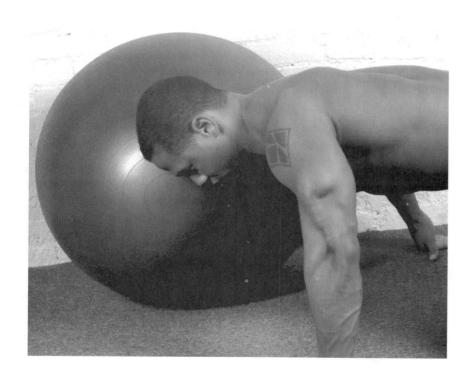

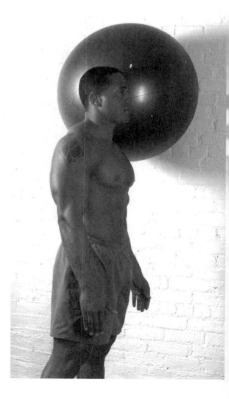

Chapter 5

POWERSCULPT

Flexibi

Training

If you're committed to getting and staying in shape, then you must make stretching an integral part of your exercise program. As we age, our joints and muscles naturally tighten. Stretching will slow this process. And if you stretch with consistency and diligence, you can even reverse it.

Whether you have been active in sports for years, are a fitness addict, or even if you've never exercised, you've developed muscle imbalances—imbalances that will, over time, create poor postural habits. Those, in turn, create wear and tear on your joints.

Stretching a body part that you feel is tight might temporarily relieve tightness, but that tightness will return if the surrounding muscles are also tight. You know the old song that goes, "the knee bone's connected to the thigh bone"? Well, stretching, like PowerSculpt training, needs to be done in synergy—not isolation. What that means is that you need to stretch your body as a unit. Of course, this isn't simple. Think of your body as if it were a guitar; to tone up and make it play well, you need to loosen the tight strings and tighten the loose strings.

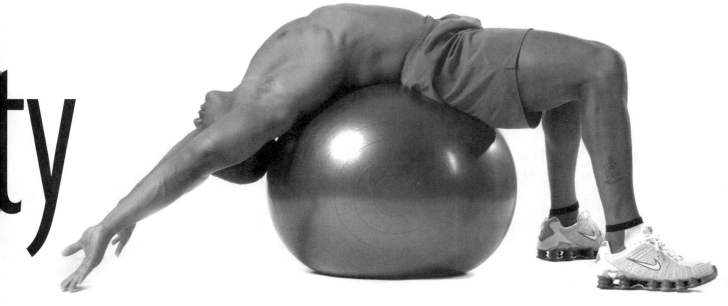

ty

There has been a slew of articles that claim stretching neither improves sports performance nor decreases the possibility of injury. The simple reason that these claims have been made is that the conventional manner of stretching—holding a stretch for 25 to 60—relaxes and elongates the muscles. This "static" stretching does nothing to prepare muscles for the quick movements required in sports, although it is cooling down after a workout or training. With this in mind, your before-workout stretches should be held at the stretch point for 1 to 2 seconds, and your after workout sessions should hold the stretch for 20 to 30 seconds.

To properly prepare to work out or to play sports you must warm up and stretch in a dynamic and rhythmic fashion: Moving in and out of a stretch briskly, holding a stretch for 2 to 3 seconds, and preferably using movements that are similar to your chosen activity.

Static stretching should be done after your activity or sport, when your muscles are thoroughly warmed. That's the perfect time to elongate and relax muscles. Stretching after a workout will also keep the muscles from quickly cooling off and becoming tighter than they were before the workout.

The Exercises

Shoulders

Keep your shoulders healthy by keeping them flexible and able to move in a full range of motion. By stretching both the shoulders and the chest you can avoid shoulder injuries.

Paul's Pro Tip

Pay attention to your breathing as you perform this and every other stretch in this section. People often hold their breath as they stretch. Proceed with caution if you have ever had a shoulder injury.

TECHNIQUE & FORM

Kneel in front of the ball and place both hands on top of it. Roll the ball forward (your chest will move toward the floor). Then roll the ball to the left and the right to stretch different muscle fibers.

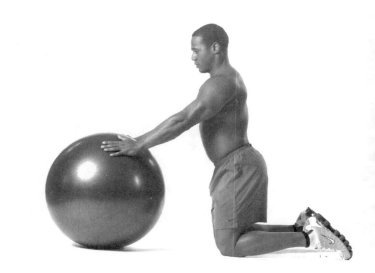

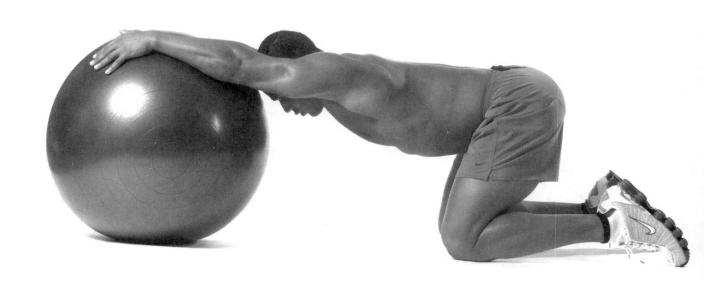

Chest I

Tight chest muscles pull the shoulders forward, creating poor posture. Stretching the chest is important to performing push-type exercise.

Paul's Pro Tip

This is also an excellent stretch for the biceps when the arm is fully extended to the side.

TECHNIQUE & FORM

Kneel on the floor with the ball on your right side. Place your right hand and forearm on the ball with your elbow bent at 90 degrees. Roll the ball backward and move your body forward so that your chest goes toward the floor. Hold 2 to 3 seconds and repeat. Repeat on both sides.

VARIATION

Extend your arm and move the ball in various positions to target different muscle fibers.

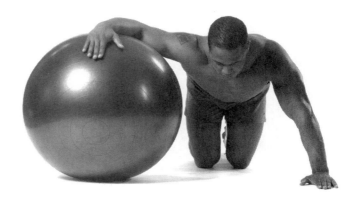

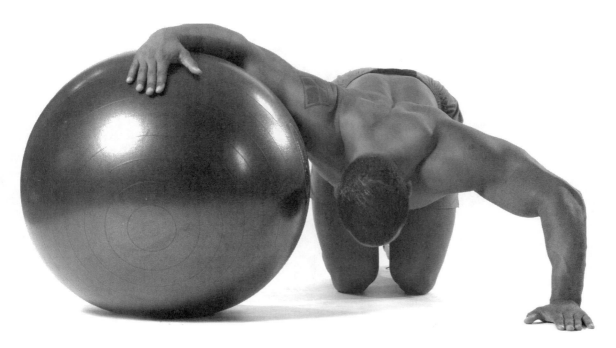

Chest II

Besides relieving daily fatigue, this stretch is great to do in the morning to relieve nighttime stiffness. It stretches and opens your chest, back, and abdominals.

TECHNIQUE & FORM
Sit on the apex of the ball, and then walk forward until the ball is supporting your lower back. Stretch out your arms to the sides. Hold 2 to 3 seconds and repeat.

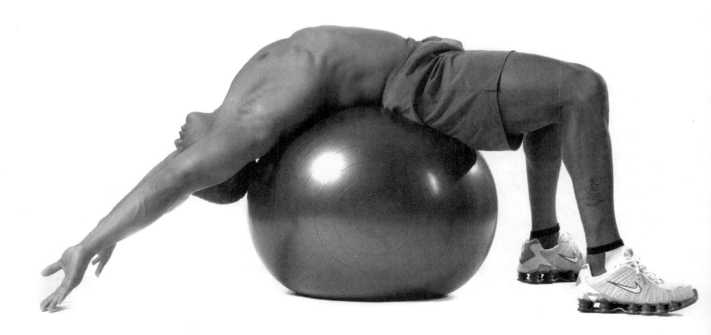

Waist

Stretching the side of the waist is essential after any abdominal training.

Paul's Pro Tip

Changing the leg position will alter the stretch from the front to the back of the waist.

TECHNIQUE & FORM

Sit on the apex of the ball, and then walk your feet forward until you're lying on top of the ball. This position stretches the *internal* and *external obliques*—the long sheet of muscle that runs down the middle of your abdomen. Hold 2 to 3 seconds. From this position, rotate to one side and reach the top arm over your head. Keep your feet wide apart for balance. Hold 2 to 3 seconds. This segment of the position stretches your waist.

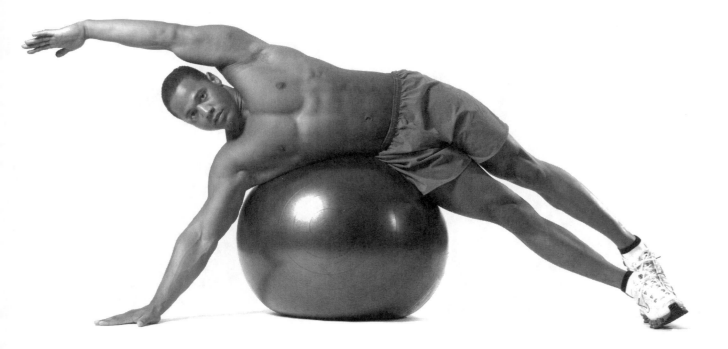

Back

Breathe deeply as you perform this stretch and you'll feel your range of motion gently increasing.

TECHNIQUE & FORM

Sit on the apex of the ball with your feet wide apart and flat on the floor. Lower your head between your knees and reach your hands toward the floor. Keep your neck and shoulders relaxed. Hold 2 to 3 seconds and repeat.

VARIATION

For a deeper stretch, wrap your arms around the inside of your calves.

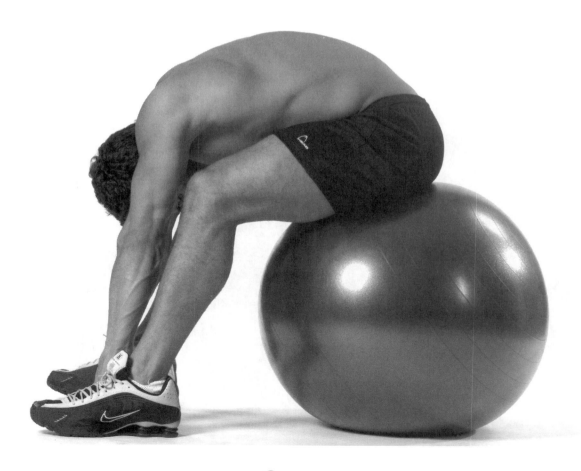

Upper Back

Changing the angle to which you apply pressure will target different muscle fibers of the back.

TECHNIQUE & FORM

Kneel in front of the ball. Place the arm that is across your chest onto the ball and gently apply downward pressure on the arm. You will feel the stretch behind the upper back and shoulder.

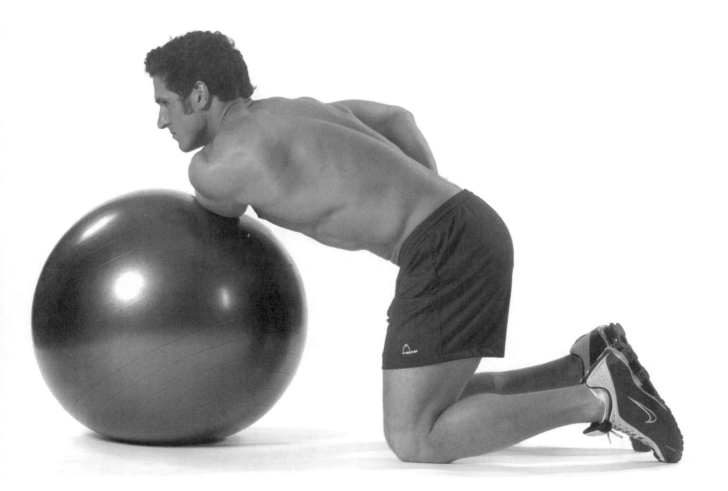

Glutes

TECHNIQUE & FORM
Place the side of your bent knee on top of the ball with the other leg extended behind you. Place both hands on the ball in front of you (as you become more flexible, drop your hands toward the floor in front of you) while bringing your chest toward the bent knee. Roll the ball around to target different muscle fibers.

This stretch is related to the pigeon pose in yoga. It not only stretches the glutes, but also opens the hips.

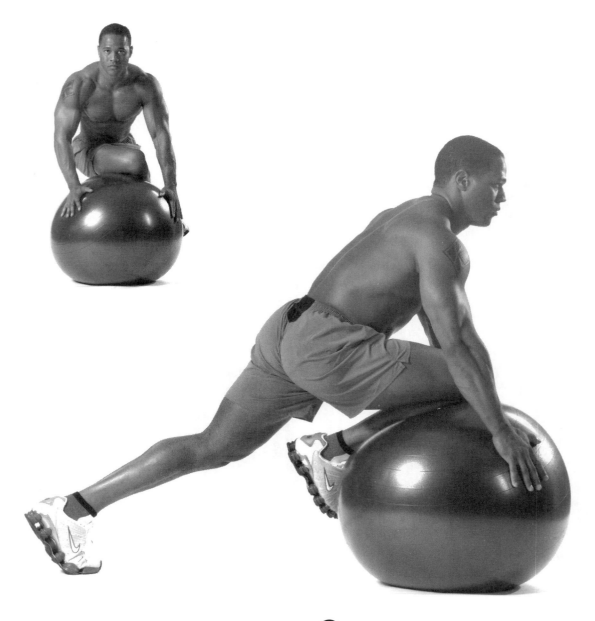

Quadriceps

TECHNIQUE & FORM

Place one knee on the floor, then place the instep of that foot on the ball. Hold 2 to 3 seconds and repeat. You'll feel the stretch in the front of your thigh.

This is really a two-part stretch: one for the front of the thigh and one for the hip flexor. It can be common to have tight thighs but loose hip flexors, or the reverse. With this stretch you can target the tight musculature.

Paul's Pro Tip

To increase this stretch and stretch the hip flexor, press your hips away from the ball.

If you're less flexible, use a smaller ball. If you're more flexible, a larger ball is more suitable.

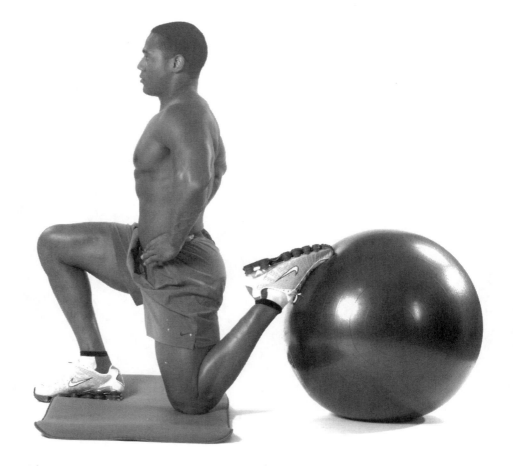

Hamstrings

The hamstrings are generally a problematic and tight muscle group. Tight hamstrings negatively affect your posture and can cause lower back pain.

Paul's Pro Tip

Maintain the arch in the lower back to target your hamstrings.

TECHNIQUE & FORM

Sit on the apex of the ball with your knees bent at a 90-degree angle and your feet flat on the floor. Push back on your heels, straighten your legs, and pull your toes toward your shins. Hold 2 to 3 seconds and repeat.

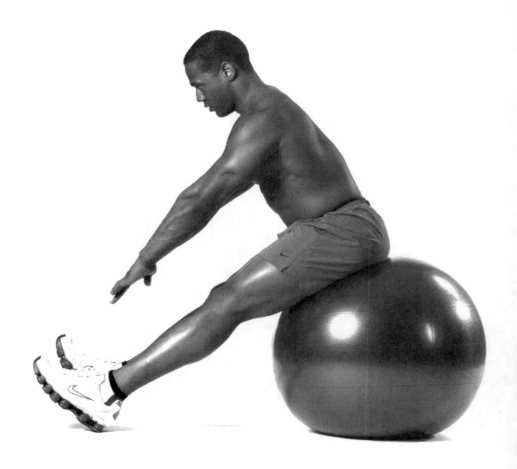

Chapter 6

POWERSCULPT
Balance

If you're walking on two feet you have at least some balance. Most individuals refuse to do any balance training because they think it's not important. It can also seem to be very tedious, boring, and quite frankly a waste of time. So why is balance important, anyway? If you participate in active pursuits that require coordination, agility, or quick footwork—think biking, hiking, ice skating, in-line skating, skiing, or windsurfing—balance training will improve your performance. Balance conditioning improves your posture. When you have good balance, you waste less energy and move more efficiently.

Even if you're not into traditional sports, you probably still walk down stairs, carry heavy loads occasionally, run for the bus, or reach for something on a high shelf. Good balance will help you with all those day-to-day tasks, too. Here's a quick way to test your balance: See how long you can stand on one foot while keeping your other leg bent. Handle that pretty well? Now do the same thing with your eyes closed. It might not be so easy.

The fitness ball is a wonderful tool for enhancing balance. Almost any exercise you do on it challenges your balance, but the poses on the following pages are especially effective for testing—and improving—your balance.

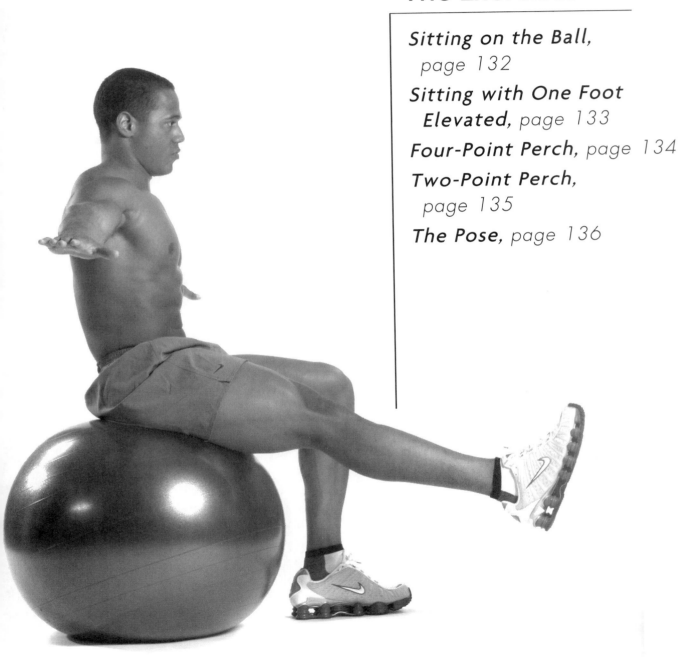

The Exercises

Sitting on the Ball

Sitting on the Ball is the first step in practicing balance.

TECHNIQUE & FORM
Sit upright on the apex of the ball with your chest high and your shoulders back.

VARIATION
Move your arms to different positions and see how your body compensates to maintain your balance.

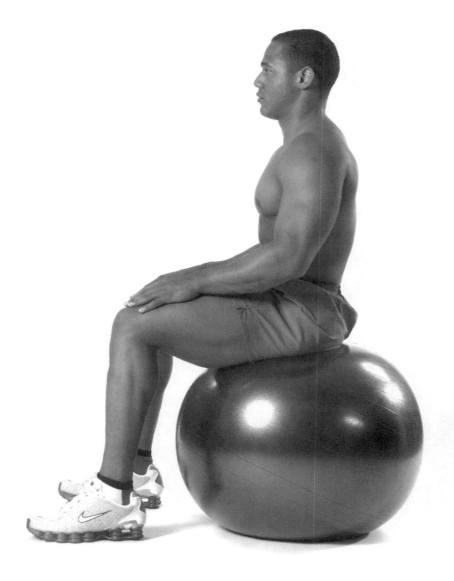

Sitting with One Foot Elevated

TECHNIQUE & FORM
Sit upright on the apex of the ball. Lift one foot a couple of inches off the floor. Change your arm position and try to maintain your balance. Switch legs and repeat.

It may look simple, but don't be surprised if you have a hard time at first.

Paul's Pro Tip

Be sure to maintain good posture—chest high, shoulders back—as you maintain balance.

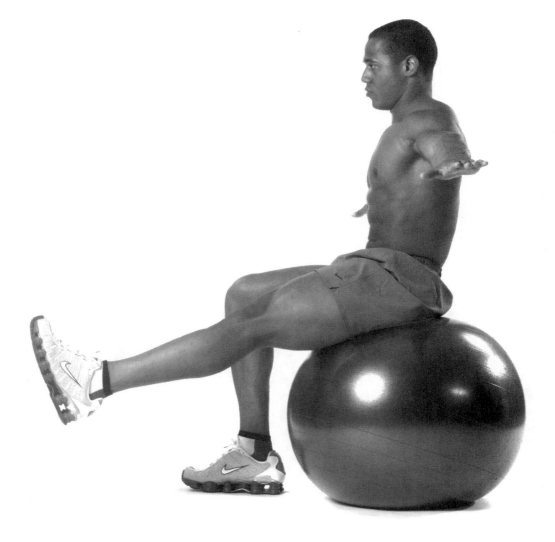

Four-Point Perch

Build up to holding this pose for 1 to 2 minutes.

Paul's Pro Tip

Keeping your insteps on the ball will give you better control. Until you're able to execute this pose, support yourself against a wall with two and then one hand.

TECHNIQUE & FORM

Stand in front of the ball. Place your hands on top of the ball and then gently allow your weight to roll you forward until your hands and knees are on the ball.

VARIATION

While in the Four-Point Perch position, extend one arm and the opposite leg. Switch and repeat.

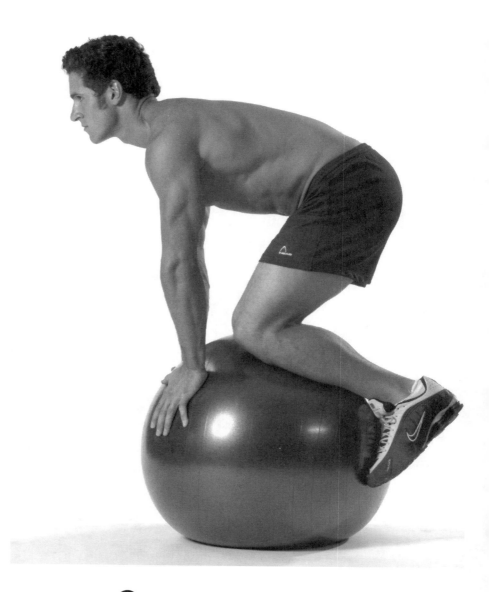

Two-Point Perch

As you do this pose, feel how much your hips and glutes need to work to stabilize your body in this position. Feel free to brace yourself against a wall until you're able to balance on your own.

Paul's Pro Tip
Once you're comfortable in this position, play catch with a partner using a tennis ball.

TECHNIQUE & FORM
From the Four Point Perch position, lift both hands off the ball. You must fully master the two-point stance position before attempting to apply weights in this position.

VARIATION: THREE-POINT PERCH
From the Four-Point Perch lift one hand off of the ball and extend the arm in front of you (as shown). Switch arms and repeat.

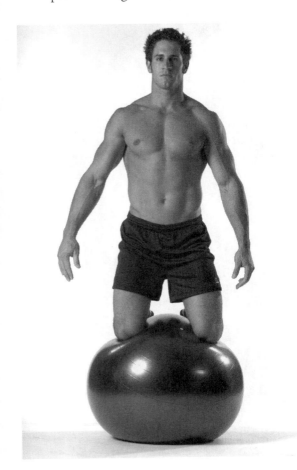

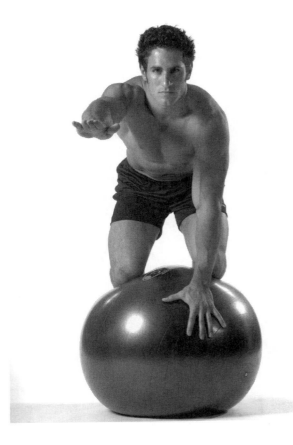

The Pose

The Pose will challenge the hip whose knee is on the ball. You will notice that one side is more stable than the other. It's a good idea to work a little extra on the unstable side.

TECHNIQUE & FORM

Start in the Four Points on the Ball position. Lift the sole of one foot onto the ball while stabilizing yourself with your hands and the opposite knee. Once you're comfortable, lift both hands off the ball.

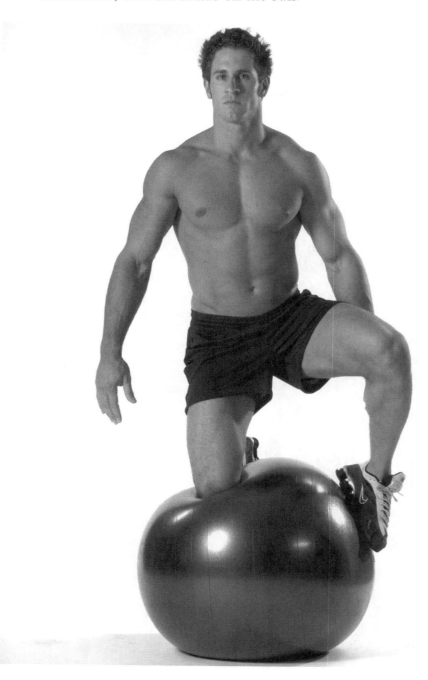

Chapter 7

The POWERSCULPT Workouts

Following the PowerSculpt Workouts sequentially —starting with Stage I—is essential for developing a safe, effective, progressive, and successful training regimen. Here are some general points to keep in mind: No two individuals are alike. The number of reps and sets are general recommendations. The workouts should be challenging—not impossible. And never, ever sacrifice form to complete a set.

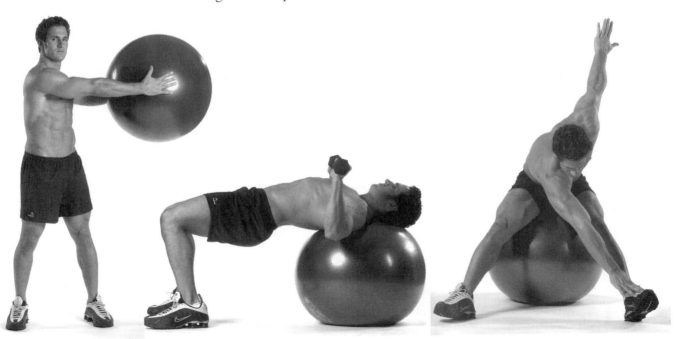

Frequently Asked Questions

"How do I find my percentage of load?"

Estimate a weight at which you can complete 10 full repetitions without losing your form through the range of motion. The weight should be challenging and you should feel that the last repetition is the last one that you will be able to complete with good form. This is known as the 10-repetition max and is one of the easier and safer methods to determine what weight you should start at.

Example: dumbbell chest press on the exercise ball. You have determined that your 10-repetition max is 100 lbs. Your chart says you should be working at 65% so that means you should select 65 lbs. as your working weight. You must also remember that because of the unstable nature of the exercise ball, it is recommended that you reduce the load by an added 20-25%. Always first perform an exercise on the ball without any load so that you acclimate yourself to the movement pattern and the necessary balance requirement.

"Why do three sets of each exercise?

We are working for the training volume (sets x reps x resistance or weight lifted) that best corresponds to developing muscular endurance in order to build a training base. Although training with a single set of 8-12 repetitions to muscular failure (i.e. you can't lift the weight another inch) will result in strength gains and bigger muscles, the neuromusculoskeletal system adapts to that stimulus and more sets are required. In some cases, a single set of 8-12 repetitions is sufficient for beginners, but it is usually not enough training volume if you have already been participating in a conditioning program.

"Would one or two sets be enough?"

It depends. If you have not done resistance training in the past, a single set might be sufficient to start with. As you continue with your program, over several months, you may find that further strength gains occur only if you increase the number of sets. Because of safety concerns I don't recommend the scheme of a single set with a load to failure unless you're an experienced weight lifter. It is important to remember that failure is when you can no longer perform the exercise with proper form.

"What is tempo?"

Tempo is the duration of each rep of a particular exercise. It dictates the length of time that your muscle is under weight bearing stimulus. For example, a 3:1:3 tempo using a biceps curl would mean lifting the weight for 3 counts, holding the top end of the movement for 1 count, then lowering for 3 counts.

"Why change the tempo of an exercise?"

Increasing the tempo increases the tension generated in the muscle that is decelerating the movement (eccentric load)—and therefore increases the strength of the tendon. The neurological reciprocal switching between agonist (acceleration) and antagonist (deceleration) must occur more quickly. A slower tempo such as 3:3:3 is best for developing the deeper postural musculature. Fast tempo of 1:0:1 with a heavier load is best for developing explosive power.

"Would splitting the workout in half and doing them alternate days be alright?"

Yes. It's perfectly fine to split your workout in half. Because of time restraints or if you're just beginning to exercise, a full program can seem overwhelming. You're better off doing less and being consistent with your workouts.

"Could I be creative with the exercise program?"

If you're an experienced exerciser, sure. But remember that when you change one of the following variables—sets, reps, and load, tempo, balance or rest interval—it often means decreasing other variables. When you make the exercise more difficult and challenging, it will stimulate the neuromusculoskeletal system. This will require the body to adapt to the ever-changing demands placed on it, which results in strength increase. It is important to first establish a base of general fitness by beginning with Phase I. Let's get started!

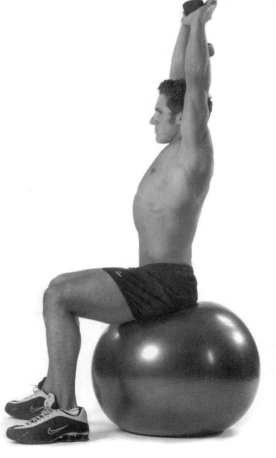

Dynamic Warm-Ups

Always begin your training with a dynamic warm-up of 8-10 minutes. Many may find that the warm-up may be a workout itself. If this is the case, begin with 10 minutes and increase 2 minutes per week until you can comfortably exercise for a total of 30 minutes. Dynamic warm-ups on the ball are excellent preparations for sports or recreational activities.

Legend

Set:	A completed number of repetitions
Reps:	The number of repetitions to complete a set
Load:	The amount of resistance
Tempo:	The pace which you move during the exercise.
BI:	Bilateral. Exercising both limbs at the same time
BW:	Body Weight
DB:	Dumbbell
RI:	Rest Interval
SS:	Split Set
UNI:	Unilateral. Exercising one limb at a time

Core Set 1

Reverse Crunch	25x	
Crunch with Rotation	25x	
Crunch	25x	
Back Extension	25x	2x

Balance Set 1

Sitting on Ball	30-60 seconds
Sitting on Ball with One Foot Elevated	30-60 seconds

Core Set 2

Lateral Crunch	25x	
Prone Crunch with Knee Curl	25x	
Abs Roll	15x	
Back Extension	25x	2x

Balance Set 2

Four-Point Perch with Hands on Floor	60-100 seconds
Four-Point Perch	60-100 seconds

Core Set 3

Prone Crunch with Knee Curl	25x	
The Pike	15x	
Prone Scissor Rotations	25x	
Back Extension	25x	2x

Balance Set 3

Two-Point Perch	60+ seconds
The Pose	60+ seconds
Two Point Cross Stance	60+ seconds

NOTE: You should do two sets of 25 back extensions each in each core set.

Phase 1: Foundation and Adaptation

WEEKS 1-4

2-3x Per Week

This stage is for anyone new to fitness ball training, whether you are a beginner or a senior. It takes roughly 4 to 6 weeks to adapt to each exercise program. This phase develops awareness of your body's balance and equilibrium. In this stage you will use light weights, higher reps, and a long tempo.

	SETS	REPS	LOAD	TEMPO	REST INTERVAL
BALANCE SET I	1-3	1-3	BW	30-60sec	<60sec
CHEST—BW					
Push-Ups	1-3	10-15	BW	3:1:3	<60sec
BACK—DB					
One-Arm Standing Rows	1-3	10-15	65%	3:1:3	<60sec
SHOULDER—DB					
Seated Lateral	1-3	10-15	65%	3:1:3	<60sec
Seated Posterior	1-3	10-15	65%	3:1:3	<60sec
Seated Anterior	1-3	10-15	65%	3:1:3	<60sec
BICEPS—DB					
Seated Biceps Curl	1-3	10-15	65%	3:1:3	<60sec
Incline Biceps Curl	1-3	10-15	65%	3:1:3	<60sec
TRICEPS—DB					
Seated Overhead Extension	1-3	10-15	65%	3:1:3	<60sec
Standing Triceps Extension	1-3	10-15	65%	3:1:3	<60sec
HAMSTRING—BW					
Hip Extensions (heels on ball, head on floor)	1-3	10-15	BW	3:3:3	<60sec
QUADS—DB					
Wall Squats	1-3	10-15	65%	3:2:3	<60sec
CALVES—DB					
Seated Calf Raise	1-3	15-20	65%	3:1:3	<60sec
Front Wall Slide	1-3	15-20	65%	3:1:3	<60sec
CORE SET I—BW	1-3	20-25	BW	3:1:3	<60sec

NOTES & OPTIONS

Increase to Balance Set 2 when you find Balance Set 1 no longer challenging.

Phase 2: Strength and Stability

WEEKS 4-8

2-3x Per Week

This phase takes into consideration that a comfort level with the ball has been developed, and begins to train to increase strength and build muscle tone. To do this, we will increase the amount of weights, quicken the tempo, and follow an increasingly difficult set of exercises.

	SETS	REPS	LOAD	TEMPO	REST INTERVAL
BALANCE SET 2	1-3	1-3	BW	30-60sec	<60sec
CHEST—BW					
Chest Press	1-3	10-12	75%	2:1:2	<60sec
Dumbbell Flies	1-3	10-12	75%	2:1:2	<60sec
BACK—DB					
One-Arm Standing Rows	1-3	10-12	75%	2:1:2	<60sec
Prone Row	1-3	10-12	75%	2:1:2	<60sec
SHOULDER—DB					
Seated Lateral	1-3	10-12	75%	2:1:2	<60sec
Seated Posterior	1-3	10-12	75%	2:1:2	<60sec
Seated Anterior	1-3	10-12	75%	2:1:2	<60sec
BICEPS—DB					
Seated Biceps Curl	1-3	10-12	75%	2:1:2	<60sec
Incline Biceps Curl	1-3	10-12	75%	2:1:2	<60sec
Preacher Curls	1-3	10-12	75%	2:1:2	<60sec
TRICEPS—DB					
Table Top Triceps Extension	1-3	10-12	75%	2:1:2	<60sec
Long Head Press	1-3	10-12	75%	2:1:2	<60sec
HAMSTRING—BW					
Double Leg Hamstring Curls	1-3	10-12	BW	2:1:2	<60sec
QUADS—DB					
Wall Squats	1-3	10-12	75%	2:1:2	<60sec
Lunge and Roll	1-3	10-12	75%	2:1:2	<60sec
CALVES—DB					
Seated Calf Raise	1-3	15-20	75%	2:1:2	<60sec
Front Wall Slide	1-3	15-20	75%	2:1:2	<60sec
CORE SET 2—BW	1-3	20-25	BW		<60sec

Phase 3: Power and Performance

WEEKS 9-12

2-3x Per Week

Phase 3 puts it all together. Once you arrive at this level, you will need heavier weights, less reps, and a quicker tempo. You will be developing power, usable in your everyday life as well as sports performance.

	SETS	REPS	LOAD	TEMPO	REST INTERVAL
BALANCE SET 3	1-3	1-3	BW	30-60sec	<60sec
CHEST—BW					
Chest Press	1-3	8-10	85%	1:1:1	<60sec
Dumbbell Flies	1-3	8-10	85%	1:1:1	<60sec
BACK—DB					
One-Arm Standing Rows	1-3	8-10	85%	1:1:1	<60sec
Prone Row	1-3	8-10	85%	1:1:1	<60sec
SHOULDER—DB					
Seated Lateral Raise	1-3	8-10	85%	1:1:1	<60sec
Reverse Fly	1-3	8-10	85%	1:1:1	<60sec
Seated Anterior Raise	1-3	8-10	85%	1:1:1	<60sec
BICEPS—DB					
Seated Biceps Curl	1-3	8-10	85%	1:1:1	<60sec
Incline Biceps Curl	1-3	8-10	85%	1:1:1	<60sec
Preacher Curls	1-3	8-10	85%	1:1:1	<60sec
TRICEPS—DB					
Tabletop Triceps Extension	1-3	8-10	85%	1:1:1	<60sec
Long Head Press	1-3	8-10	85%	1:1:1	<60sec
HAMSTRING—BW					
Double Leg Hamstring Curls	1-3	8-10	BW	2:1:2	<60sec
QUADS—DB					
Wall Squats	1-3	8-10	85%	1:1:1	<60sec
Lunge and Roll	1-3	8-10	85%	1:1:1	<60sec
CALVES—DB					
Seated Calf Raise	1-3	8-10	85%	1:1:1	<60sec
Front Wall Slide	1-3	8-10	85%	1:1:1	<60sec
CORE SET 3—BW	1-3	20-25	BW		<60sec

PowerSculpt Blast Circuit

If you're a person that doesn't have lots of time but understands the importance of strength training, then this workout is for you. The PowerSculpt Blast Circuit is a quick and intensive body-strengthening program. You choose one body part per day and exercise it to fatigue. For example, you will exercise five days a week, concentrating on a select body part each day. The Balance Set and Ab Blast are optional to include in your workout. Be sure to include a good warm-up before (and stretch after) your circuit.

If a full body circuit is what your enjoy then select one exercise for each body part, and do one set of each. The less you rest between sets the more cardio benefit you will receive. Do 1-3 sets, and only follow this regime five days a week.

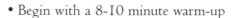

- Begin with a 8-10 minute warm-up
- Choose a level of weight that is challenging but not impossible.
- Always remember form first.
- To receive the most in cardio and fat burning benefits rest as little as possible between sets.
- Try increasing the amount of weight or reps done by 5% every 2 weeks.
- At the end of 6 weeks you will have increased the amount of weight your lifting by 10%.
- Begin weeks 6 through 10 by reducing the weight lifted by 10% and increase the reps by 10%.
- After week 10, try changing the variables. Changing the reps, weight, and tempo on a regular basis will force your body to adapt. This will make you stronger, leaner and more toned.
- Do 2-3 minutes of stretching the body part exercised.

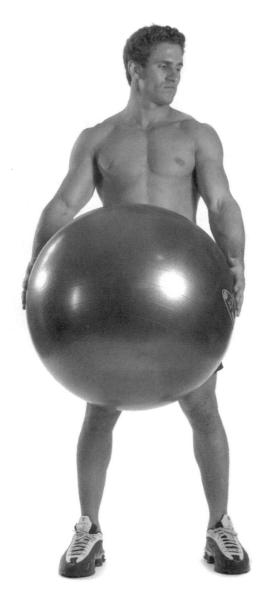